Computer-aided vaccine design

Published by Woodhead Publishing Limited, 2013

Woodhead Publishing Series in Biomedicine

1 Practical leadership for biopharmaceutical executives
J. Y. Chin
2 Outsourcing biopharma R&D to India
P. R. Chowdhury
3 Matlab® in bioscience and biotechnology
L. Burstein
4 Allergens and respiratory pollutants
Edited by M. A. Williams
5 Concepts and techniques in genomics and proteomics
N. Saraswathy and P. Ramalingam
6 An introduction to pharmaceutical sciences
J. Roy
7 Patently innovative: How pharmaceutical firms use emerging patent law to extend monopolies on blockbuster drugs
R. A. Bouchard
8 Therapeutic protein drug products: Practical approaches to formulation in the laboratory, manufacturing and the clinic
Edited by B. K. Meyer
9 A biotech manager's handbook: A practical guide
Edited by M. O'Neill and M. H. Hopkins
10 Clinical research in Asia: Opportunities and challenges
U. Sahoo
11 Therapeutic antibody engineering: Current and future advances driving the strongest growth area in the pharma industry
W. R. Strohl and L. M. Strohl
12 Commercialising the stem cell sciences
O. Harvey
13 Biobanks: Patents or open science?
A. De Robbio

14 Human papillomavirus infections: From the laboratory to clinical practice
F. Cobo
15 Annotating new genes: From *in silico* screening to experimental validation
S. Uchida
16 Open-source software in life science research: Practical solutions in the pharmaceutical industry and beyond
Edited by L. Harland and M. Forster
17 Nanoparticulate drug delivery: A perspective on the transition from laboratory to market
V. Patravale, P. Dandekar and R. Jain
18 Bacterial cellular metabolic systems: Metabolic regulation of a cell system with ^{13}C-metabolic flux analysis
K. Shimizu
19 Contract research and manufacturing services (CRAMS) in India: The business, legal, regulatory and tax environment
M. Antani and G. Gokhale
20 Bioinformatics for biomedical science and clinical applications
K-H. Liang
21 Deterministic versus stochastic modelling in biochemistry and systems biology
P. Lecca, I. Laurenzi and F. Jordan
22 Protein folding *in silico*: Protein folding versus protein structure prediction
I. Roterman
23 Computer-aided vaccine design
J. C. Tong and S. Ranganathan
24 An introduction to biotechnology
W. T. Godbey
25 RNA interference: Therapeutic developments
T. Novobrantseva, P. Ge and G. Hinkle
26 Patent litigation in the pharmaceutical and biotechnology industries
G. Morgan
27 Clinical research in paediatric psychopharmacology: A practical guide
P. Auby
28 The application of SPC in the pharmaceutical and biotechnology industries
T. Cochrane

29 Ultrafiltration for bioprocessing
H. Lutz
30 Therapeutic risk management of medicines
A. K. Banerjee and S. Mayall
31 21st century quality management and good management practices: Value added compliance for the pharmaceutical and biotechnology industry
S. Williams
32 Sterility, sterilisation and sterility assurance for pharmaceuticals
T. Sandle
33 CAPA in the pharmaceutical and biotech industries: How to implement an effective nine step programme
J. Rodriguez
34 Process validation for the production of biopharmaceuticals: Principles and best practice
A. R. Newcombe and P. Thillaivinayagalingam
35 Clinical trial management: An overview
U. Sahoo and D. Sawant
36 Impact of regulation on drug development
H. Guenter Hennings
37 Lean biomanufacturing
N. J. Smart
38 Marine enzymes for biocatalysis
Edited by A. Trincone
39 Ocular transporters and receptors in the eye: Their role in drug delivery
A. K. Mitra
40 Stem cell bioprocessing: For cellular therapy, diagnostics and drug development
T. G. Fernandes, M. M. Diogo and J. M. S. Cabral
41 Oral delivery of insulin
T. A. Sonia and Chandra P. Sharma
42 Fed-batch fermentation: A practical guide to scalable recombinant protein production in *Escherichia coli*
G. G. Moulton and T. Vedvick
43 The funding of biopharmaceutical research and development
D. R. Williams
44 Formulation tools for pharmaceutical development
Edited by J. E. A. Diaz

45 Drug-biomembrane interaction studies: The application of calorimetric techniques
Edited by R. Pignatello

46 Orphan drugs: Understanding the rare drugs market
E. Hernberg-Ståhl

47 Nanoparticle-based approaches to targeting drugs for severe diseases
J. L. Arias

48 Successful biopharmaceutical operations: Driving change
C. Driscoll

49 Electroporation-based therapies for cancer: From basics to clinical applications
Edited by R. Sundararajan

50 Transporters in drug discovery and development: Detailed concepts and best practice
Y. Lai

51 The life-cycle of pharmaceuticals in the environment
R. Braund and B. Peake

52 Computer-aided applications in pharmaceutical technology
Edited by J. Djuris

53 From plant genomics to plant biotechnology
Edited by P. Poltronieri, N. Burbulis and C. Fogher

54 Bioprocess engineering: An introductory engineering and life science approach
K. G. Clarke

55 Quality assurance problem solving and training strategies for success in the pharmaceutical and life science industries
G. Welty

56 Advancement in carrier based drug delivery
S. K. Jain and A. Jain

57 Gene therapy: Potential applications of nanotechnology
S. Nimesh

58 Controlled drug delivery: The role of self-assembling multi-task excipients
M. Mateescu

59 *In silico* protein design
C. M. Frenz

60 Bioinformatics for computer science: Foundations in modern biology
K. Revett

Woodhead Publishing Series in Biomedicine: Number 23

Computer-aided vaccine design

Joo Chuan Tong and
Shoba Ranganathan

WP
WOODHEAD
PUBLISHING

Oxford Cambridge Philadelphia New Delhi

Published by Woodhead Publishing Limited, 2013

Woodhead Publishing Limited, 80 High Street, Sawston, Cambridge, CB22 3HJ, UK
www.woodheadpublishing.com
www.woodheadpublishingonline.com

Woodhead Publishing, 1518 Walnut Street, Suite 1100, Philadelphia,
PA 19102–3406, USA

Woodhead Publishing India Private Limited, G-2, Vardaan House, 7/28 Ansari Road,
Daryaganj, New Delhi – 110002, India
www.woodheadpublishingindia.com

First published in 2013 by Woodhead Publishing Limited
ISBN: 978–1–907568–41–1 (print); ISBN 978–1–908818–41–6 (online)
Woodhead Publishing Series in Biomedicine ISSN 2050-0289 (print);
ISSN 2050-0297 (online)

British Library Cataloguing-in-Publication Data: A catalogue record for this book is available from the British Library.

Library of Congress Control Number: 2013936016

Typeset by RefineCatch Limited, Bungay, Suffolk
Printed in the UK and USA

Contents

Published by Woodhead Publishing Limited, 2013

Published by Woodhead Publishing Limited, 2013

List of figures

Published by Woodhead Publishing Limited, 2013

Published by Woodhead Publishing Limited, 2013

Published by Woodhead Publishing Limited, 2013

Published by Woodhead Publishing Limited, 2013

List of abbreviations

ACC	accuracy
ACD	Available Chemical Directory
ADME/Tox	absorption, distribution, metabolism, excretion and toxicity
ANN	artificial neural network
APC	antigen presenting cell
A_{ROC}	area under the receiver operating characteristic curve
β_2m	β_2-microglobulin
BCG	Bacillus Calmette-Guérin
BCNF	Boyce–Codd normal form
BEID	B cell epitope interaction database
BIMAS	BioInformatics and Molecular Analysis Section
BLAST	Basic Local Alignment Search Tool
BLOSUM	BLOck SUbstitution Matrix
BMRB	Biological Magnetic Resonance Data Bank
CD4	cluster of differentiation 4
CD8	cluster of differentiation 8
CED	Conformational Epitope Database
CHIKV	Chikungunya virus
CIB	Center for Information Biology
CIF	Crystallographic Information File
CLL	Chronic Lymphocytic Leukemia
CMC	Comprehensive Medicinal Chemistry
CoMSIA	Comparative molecular similarity index analysis

DDBJ	DNA Data Bank of Japan
d_N	non-synonymous substitution
d_S	synonymous substitution
EBI	European Bioinformatics Institute
EMBL	European Molecular Biology Laboratory
ENA	European Nucleotide Archive
ER	endoplasmic reticulum or entity-relationship
ERAAP	ER aminopeptidase associated with antigen processing
EST	expressed sequence tag
ESTDAB	European Searchable Tumour Cell-Line Database
FAO	Food and Agriculture Organization
Fc region	fragment crystallizable region
FDA	Food and Drug Administration
GSS	genome survey sequence
HBA	hydrogen bond acceptor
HBD	hydrogen bond donor
HCV	hepatitis C virus
HIV	human immunodeficiency virus
HLA	human leukocyte antigen
HMM	hidden Markov model
HPLC	high-performance liquid chromatography
IEDB	Immune Epitope Database
IFBC	International Food Biotechnology Council
IFN	interferon
Ig	immunoglobulin
Ii	invariant chain
ILIS	International Life Sciences Institute
InChI	International Chemical Identifier
INSDC	International Nucleotide Sequence Database Collaboration
IPD	Immuno Polymorphism Database
kNN	*k*-Nearest-Neighbor

Published by Woodhead Publishing Limited, 2013

LMP-2	low molecular weight proteins (LMP)-2
LMP-7	low molecular weight proteins (LMP)-7
logP	n-octanol/water partition coefficient
MBL	mannan-binding lectin
MC	Markov chain
MECL	multicatalytic endopeptidase complex
MEDLINE	Medical Literature Analysis and Retrieval System Online
MeSH	Medical Subject Headings
MHC	major histocompatibility complex
MI	mutual information
MIF	molecular interaction field
MIIC	MHC class II compartment
ML	maximum likelihood
MPID-T	MHC-peptide interaction database-TR
MW	molecular weight
NAR	Nucleic Acids Research
NCBI	National Center for Biotechnology Information
NCI	National Cancer Institute
NIAID	National Institute of Allergy and Infectious Diseases
NIG	National Institute of Genetics
NIH	National Institute of Health
NLM	National Library of Medicine
NME	new molecular entities
NMR	nuclear magnetic resonance
PAIN	Pan Assay Interference Compound
PAM	Percent Accepted Mutation
PCA	principal component analysis
PDB	protein data bank
PDBe	PDB Europe
PDBj	PDB Japan
PIR	Protein Information Resource

PSA	polar surface area
QSAR	quantitative structure–affinity relationship
RCSB	Research Collaboratory for Structural Bioinformatics
RMSD	root mean square deviation
RPI	related proteins of the immune system
SARS-CoV	severe acute respiratory syndrome coronavirus
scFv	single chain Fragment variable
SDF	Structure Data Format
SE	sensitivity
SIB	Swiss Institute of Bioinformatics
SLN	SYBYL Line Notation
SMILES	Simplified Molecular Input Line Entry Specification
SMM	stabilized matrix method
SP	specificity
STS	sequence-tagged sites
SVM	support vector machine
TAP	transporter associated with antigen processing
TCR	T cell receptor
TPSA	topological polar surface area
TR	T cell receptor
TrEMBL	Translated EMBL
UniMES	UniProt Metagenomic and Environmental Sequences database
UniParc	UniProt Archive
UniProtKB	UniProt Knowledgebase
UniRef	UniProt Reference Clusters
USPTO	United States Patent and Trademark Office proteins
WDI	World Drug Index
WGS	whole genome shotgun

Published by Woodhead Publishing Limited, 2013

WHO	World Health Organization
WOMBAT	World of Molecular BioAcTivity
wwPDB	Worldwide Protein Data Bank

Published by Woodhead Publishing Limited, 2013

About the authors

Joo Chuan Tong

Joo Chuan graduated with a BSc (Honors) in Computer Science from the School of Computing, National University of Singapore (NUS) in 2002 and a PhD in Biochemistry from the Department of Biochemistry, Yong Loo Lin School of Medicine, NUS in 2007. In 2005, he joined the Institute for Infocomm Research (I2R) under the Agency for Science, Technology and Research (A*STAR) to work on a National Institutes of Health (NIH)-funded project under Prof Vladimir Brusic. He went on to head the biomedical informatics group at I2R from 2007 to 2012. In 2009, he served as a member of the inaugural Senior Innovation Advisory Board of Pfizer Inc., the world's largest research-based pharmaceutical company, providing strategic advice to the executive leadership team at their world headquarters in New York, USA. Since 2009, he has served as an Adjunct Assistant Professor at the Department of Biochemistry, Yong Loo Lin School of Medicine, NUS. Joo Chuan is currently the Treasurer of the Asia-Pacific Bioinformatics Network and Faculty Advisor to the International Society for Computational Biology Regional Student Group (ISCB-RSG) in Singapore. He is also the past president of the Association for Medical and Bio-Informatics, Singapore (AMBIS).

Joo Chuan has had a highly decorated career in computational biology, he and his team having won more than 20 international, national, and institutional awards over

Published by Woodhead Publishing Limited, 2013

the past five years. He was a recipient of the prestigious MIT TR35 Award in 2008 for the world's top 35 science and technology innovators under the age of 35 for his work on computer-aided vaccine design. In 2009, he received the Singapore Youth Award (Science & Technology), the nation's highest accolade for youth excellence below the age of 35, for his work on computational immunology. In 2012, he was named a Young Global Leader by the World Economic Forum, for the potential of his work in shaping the global future. His current areas of research interest include computational immunology, computational epigenetics, combinatorial library design, and computational modeling of biological systems.

Shoba Ranganathan

Shoba is one of the few principal researchers in the world working in several key areas of bioinformatics, to understand biological systems using computational approaches. She has extensive experience and expertise in different aspects of computational biology, ranging from metabolites and small molecules to biochemical networks and pathway analysis. She has developed several novel databases (DEDB, MPID, MPID-T, OMIA, SPdb, XPro, CMKb), computational methodologies (MGAlign, MHC-peptide docking protocol, splicing subgraph identification and mapping, chemoinformatics analysis), web services (MGAlignIt, SDPMOD, ASGS, CASVM, ESTExplorer, EST2Secretome), and grid-based bioinformatics applications (APBioBox, APKnoPPIX). Her current areas of research include structure-based immunogenic epitope prediction, host–parasite interactions, secretome analysis, and graph theoretical approaches to study the phenomenon of alternative splicing.

Shoba has worked in the area of bioinformatics, as an academic researcher and teacher and also as a consultant to

Published by Woodhead Publishing Limited, 2013

industry. Shoba's achievements in the field of bioinformatics research and teaching have contributed to her election to the Board of Directors of the International Society for Computational Biology (ISCB), where she served as the first Australasian Director (2003–5). She is currently the President, Asia-Pacific Bioinformatics Network (APBioNet); Council Member, International Immunomics Society; and Steering Committee Member, Bioinformatics Australia. She has helped organize international conferences in Bioinformatics, including the Intelligent Systems in Molecular Biology (ISMB) conferences, International Conference in Bioinformatics (InCoB), the Asia-Pacific Bioinformatics Conference, and the Genome Informatics Workshop. She also pioneered the Workshops on Education in Bioinformatics (WEB), now an ISCB Special Interest Group meeting, and the Workshops on Education in Bioinformatics and Computational Biology (WEBCB) as InCoB satellite meetings. She reviews grant applications from Australia, USA, UK, Hong Kong, and Spain. She is on the editorial board of leading bioinformatics journals such as *Briefings in Bioinformatics, BMC Bioinformatics, Immunome Research, Evolutionary Biology*, and *BMC Supplements*. She was also awarded a UNESCO Chair in Biodiversity Informatics for linking genomes to phenomes. Shoba's main contributions to APBioNet are the affiliation with ISCB; establishing InCoB as a premier bioinformatics conference in the region; pioneering the publication of the best InCoB papers as *BMC Bioinformatics/Genomics* supplements; and obtaining research grants from IDRC, Canada and education grants from IUBMB. Her contribution to APBioNet will be her experience in bioinformatics education, governance, and conference organization. She is also spearheading the 100 BioDatabases project, which will conform to the MIABi standards proposed at InCoB2009.

Published by Woodhead Publishing Limited, 2013

Preface

Vaccination has its roots in 1796, when an English scientist by the name of Edward Jenner inoculated James Phipps, his gardener's eight-year-old son, with material from the cowpox blisters of the hand of Sarah Nelmes, a milkmaid infected with cowpox from a cow named Blossom. Jenner went on to show that by inoculation with cowpox people became immune to smallpox, and that protective cowpox could be effectively inoculated from person to person. This work laid the foundation for the design of modern vaccines, and Blossom's hide is now enshrined in the library of St George's medical school to commemorate the pioneer of smallpox vaccination and the father of immunology. Since then, vaccines have changed the world and saved the lives of millions of people worldwide.

First generation vaccines contain killed or inactivated micro-organisms in their entirety. Louis Pasteur was the first person to introduce the use of artificially attenuated viruses in vaccines, first in chicken cholera vaccine in the 1870s and anthrax vaccine for sheep and cattle in 1881, followed by the rabies vaccine for humans in 1885. Such vaccines have been shown to be capable of inducing killer/helper T cell immunity as well as antibody-mediated immunity. Despite their successes, vaccines made using live attenuated pathogens are risky, as the weakened pathogens may undergo secondary mutations in the body and become virulent again. Moreover, they may also cause disease in immunocompromised vaccine recipients. While killed vaccines do not present these risks,

Published by Woodhead Publishing Limited, 2013

their efficacy varies greatly, as the natural conformation of the pathogens may be altered and hence affect their ability to present to antigen presenting cells. Second generation vaccines are vaccines that contain fragments of pathogens (i.e. defined protein antigens) capable of stimulating the immune system. Such subunit vaccines are particularly attractive as they could offer the effectiveness of live attenuated vaccines without their associated risks. Third generation vaccines adopt a similar strategy, and comprise genetically engineered pathogen DNA capable of producing protein antigens that can induce immune responses. A major challenge with both second and third generation vaccines is to identify the essential antigens that best stimulate immune responses. This is difficult due to the great diversity of the immune system's components, the complexity of its regulatory pathways, and the huge variability of pathogen products.

In the last two decades, advances in bioinformatics technology have changed the face of vaccine research. Computational methods of data management, data mining, pattern recognition, and visualization are now routinely used to help advance vaccine discovery efforts. This book aims to serve as an introductory book as well as a reference book covering the central resources, tools, and techniques necessary for a successful computer-aided vaccine design campaign. A large number of biological and chemical databases are now available in the public domain. Harnessing the power of these databases requires expert knowledge and advanced navigation skills. The ever growing quantities of biological and chemical data require increasingly sophisticated and powerful tools for analysis and visualization. The topics discussed span multiple areas including computer science, epidemiology, immunology, machine learning, mathematics, and statistics.

The book is written both for students and researchers in molecular biology who would like to understand the fundamentals of the bioinformatics software or methods that are essential in a computer-aided vaccine design campaign, and for computer scientists who would like to know more about the biology of key topics in this rapidly growing field. By reading this book, the first group of readers should gain a better understanding of the strengths and weaknesses of available methods, thereby becoming more capable in selecting the right software to facilitate the analysis of results; while the second group of readers should become more informed of the biological basis underlying this field, thereby allowing them to design more sophisticated computational algorithms for vaccine discovery.

The book material and treatment reflect our personal perspectives in the field of computer-aided vaccine design. A challenge in writing this book has been to find the right combination of contents such that the materials are interesting and relevant to both groups of readers with contrasting backgrounds. We have done this by focusing on the concepts of the methods and algorithms, and how they can be applied in the study of key biological processes. In order to facilitate the explanation of key concepts, we have included numerous examples that illustrate the basic concepts and ideas. We have also included a bibliographic section at the end of each chapter that points to relevant resources and original research papers for readers who would like to learn more about the subject. A large number of algorithms have emerged over the last few years, many of which have contributed greatly to the development of this rapidly growing field. We would have liked to describe all of them in detail, but some of these methods had to be omitted for us to stay within the size limit of the book. In cases where we are not able to delve more deeply into a subject topic, we have tried to provide ample references to the readers for possible extension outside the context of this book.

We assume that the reader has a basic knowledge of biology, mathematics and computer science. Short introductions to the central concepts of immunology, infectious diseases, and bioinformatics are included to help readers understand the biological basis of computer-aided vaccine design, core concepts in computer science, and some basic mathematics. We also include in the list of abbreviations the common terms and terminologies used in the field, and recommend readers check out the list before reading the book.

Published by Woodhead Publishing Limited, 2013

1

MHC and T cell responses

DOI: 10.1533/9781908818416.1

Abstract: The major histocompatibility complex (MHC) molecules of classes I and II, coded by the human leukocyte antigen (HLA) genes on chromosome 6, are cell surface glycoproteins that play a major role in T cell-mediated immune recognition. Class I molecules are found on the surface of virtually all nucleated cells in humans, except neurons, and are involved in detection of viral infections in cells. Class II molecules are limited to specific antigen presenting cells. In both cases, T cell antigen recognition is triggered by the MHC presenting a short antigenic peptide fragment which binds to a specific T cell receptor (TCR) on the surface of T cells. In this chapter, we survey the nature of the MHC molecules and their roles in cell-mediated immune responses. The genetic organizations of the MHC class I and II molecules, their structures and functions are described.

Key words: major histocompatibility complex, human leukocyte antigen, T cell, T cell receptor, antigen presenting cell, cell-mediated immunity.

Published by Woodhead Publishing Limited, 2013

1.1 Genetic organization of the MHC

The major histocompatibility complex (MHC) molecules are cell surface glycoproteins that play a central role in T cell-mediated immune recognition. The MHC genes in humans, termed human leukocyte antigen (HLA), are found on chromosome 6. Today, HLA is organized into three major genetic regions or loci designated class I, II and III. Class III genes primarily encode components of the serum complement system. Class I and class II loci, on the other hand, encode a number of highly polymorphic cell-surface proteins responsible for antigen presentation. The HLA class I locus is subdivided into HLA-A, -B, and -C subregions, each encoding class I α chain genes. The class II HLA locus, HLA-D, is subdivided into at least six subregions, namely HLA-DR, -DQ, -DP, -DX, -DO, and -DZ. The class I and class II genes are highly polymorphic genes in the human genome; for some of these genes, over 200 allelic variants have been identified. HLA specificities are identified by an identifier for locus and a number (e.g. A1, DR4, and DQ5) and the haplotypes are identified by individual specificities. Specificities that are defined by genomic analysis are names beginning with an identifier for the locus followed by a four-digit code (e.g. A*0101, Cw*0401, and DRB1*0503). Despite considerable MHC polymorphism, a single individual expresses a finite number of MHC alleles and is heterozygous for each MHC gene in humans. The work discussed here focuses on MHC molecules that are responsible for antigen presentation. Therefore, the use of MHC for the rest of the text is restricted to only the class I and class II genes.

Published by Woodhead Publishing Limited, 2013

1.2 MHC structure

All MHC molecules share certain structural characteristics that are critical for their role in peptide display and recognition by T cells. T cell recognition of antigen is said to be MHC restricted, as T cell receptors (TCRs) will only bind to fragments of antigen that are associated with products of the MHC. Each MHC molecule contains an extracellular peptide-binding cleft which is composed of paired α-helices resting on a floor consisting of an eight-stranded anti-parallel β-sheet. This portion of the MHC molecule binds antigenic peptides for display to T cells, and the TCRs possess a complementary shape that will interact with the displayed peptide and with the helices of the MHC molecules. The amino acid residues located in and around this cleft are highly polymorphic and they are responsible for the different peptide binding specificities among different MHC alleles. A non-polymorphic determinant on the MHC molecules acts as the binding site for the T cell co-receptor molecules CD4 and CD8. CD4 and CD8 are expressed on distinct subpopulations of mature T cells and, together with the antigen receptors, participate in the recognition of antigen. CD8 binds selectively to class I MHC molecules, and CD4 binds to class II MHC molecules. Hence, $CD8^+$ T cells recognize only peptides displayed by class I molecules, and $CD4^+$ T cells recognize only peptides presented by class II molecules. Most $CD8^+$ T cells function as cytotoxic T cells and $CD4^+$ cells are helper cells.

MHC class I molecules are ternary complexes composed of a heavy glycosylated transmembrane protein non-covalently linked to a smaller polypeptide β_2-microglobulin (β_2m). The complete molecule has four globular domains: three formed by the heavy chain (α_1, α_2, α_3) and one by β_2m, as shown in Figure 1.1. Both the α_1 and α_2 domains adopt a

Published by Woodhead Publishing Limited, 2013

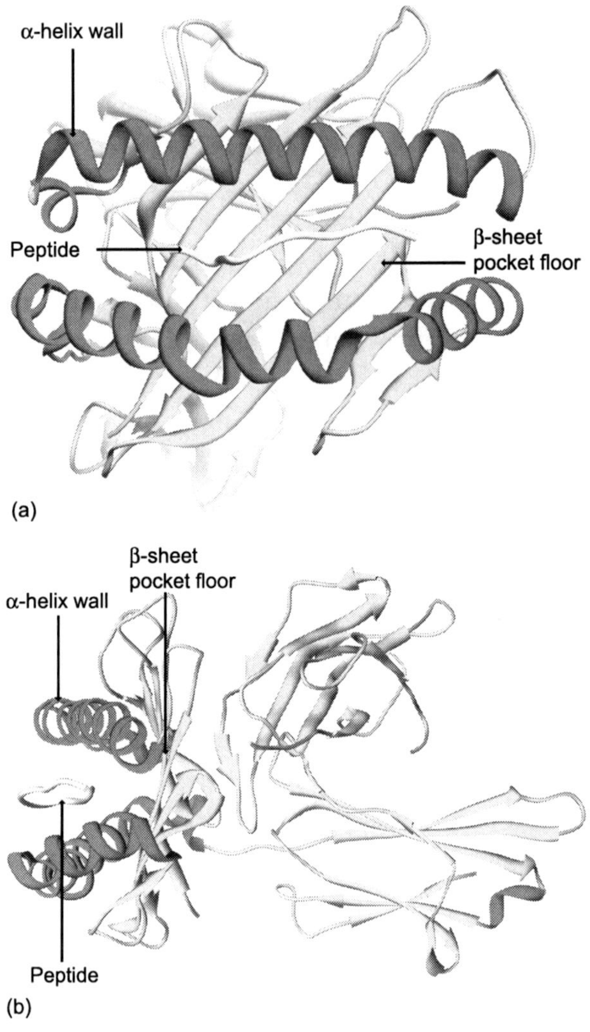

Figure 1.1 Schematic of MHC class I structure. (a) Front view of a class I molecule in complex with antigenic peptide based on X-ray crystallographic structure. (b) Side view of the same molecule clearly showing the anatomy of the peptide-binding cleft formed by α-helices sitting on a platform of a β-sheet

Published by Woodhead Publishing Limited, 2013

similar structure: starting from the N-terminus, each region of the chain forms four anti-parallel β-strands followed by a helical region across the β-strands on one side of the β-sheet. The two domains associate in such a way that their β-sheets are hydrogen-bonded to each other, forming a platform of a continuous eight-stranded anti-parallel β-sheet. The β-sheet is relatively flat with a small propeller twist. The sides of this cleft are formed by two α-helices, one from α_1 and one from α_2. It is within this cleft that antigen fragments are held and presented to T cells. The α_3 domain consists of a transmembrane segment and a short cytoplasmic tail that anchors the molecule in the membrane.

MHC class II molecules are also transmembrane glycoproteins, consisting of two polypeptide chains (α, β) held together by non-covalent interactions. Similarly to class I MHC, the complete class II MHC molecule has four globular domains, two on each chain (α_1, α_2, β_1, β_2). The α_1 and β_1 domains mimic the class I α_1 and α_2 domains in forming a peptide-binding groove bounded by two α-helices and a β-sheet floor (Figure 1.2).

1.3 MHC function

The class I MHC-restricted antigen processing and presentation pathway provides a sophisticated surveillance mechanism aimed at detecting viral infections in cells. MHC class I molecules are synthesized in the endoplasmic reticulum (ER) and are present on the surface of virtually all nucleated cells, except neurons, in humans. Their function is to bind peptides derived from endogenous antigens within the cell, transport them to the cell surface, and present the bound peptide ligands to cytotoxic T cells through the TCR and CD8. Most class I peptide ligands are derived from proteins

Published by Woodhead Publishing Limited, 2013

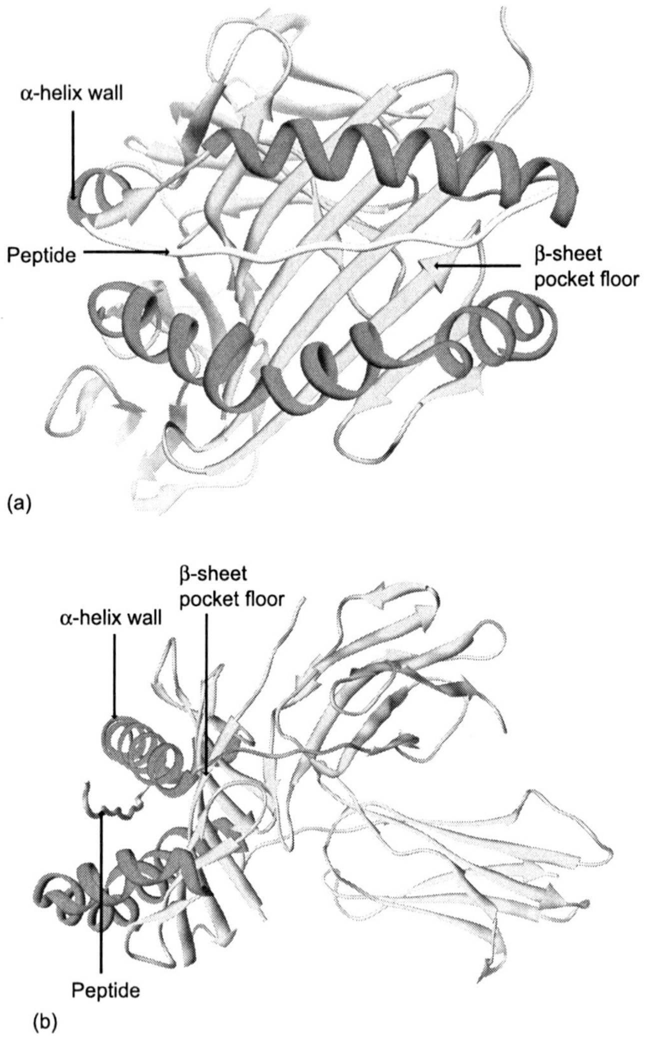

Figure 1.2 Schematic of MHC class II structure. (a) Front view of a MHC class II molecule in complex with antigenic peptide extending out of the binding cleft based on X-ray crystallographic structure. (b) Side view of the same molecule showing the anatomy of the peptide-binding cleft formed by α-helices sitting on a platform of a β-sheet

Published by Woodhead Publishing Limited, 2013

that are degraded by proteasomes. The proteasome has broad substrate specificity and can generate a wide variety of peptides from cytosolic proteins. Exposure of cells to interferon (IFN)-γ induces the synthesis of three proteolytic proteasome subunits – low molecular weight proteins (LMP)-2 and LMP-7 and multicatalytic endopeptidase complex (MECL)-1 – which are incorporated into an alternative form of proteasome, called an immunoproteasome, displacing the constitutive subunits β1, β2, and β5, respectively. At the present time, it remains unclear how the products of such endopeptidase activity are related to the final MHC class I ligands. One possibility is that the proteasomes directly produce peptides of appropriate size. Alternatively, the proteasomes may generate longer peptides that require further processing. It is also possible that two short non-continuous peptide fragments can be fused together to create the final class I ligand via post-translational protein splicing. In any case, the majority of these peptides are transported from the cytosol into the ER by the transporter associated with antigen processing (TAP). TAP consists of two structurally related subunits, which interact to form a functional peptide-transporting complex. Before peptide translocation by TAP, peptides bind to the membrane-proximal, cytosolic surface of TAP1/TAP2 complexes. Hydrolysis of ATP results in peptide translocation into the ER lumen. Within the ER lumen, precursor peptides may be further trimmed by an ER-resident aminopeptidase ERAAP (ER aminopeptidase associated with antigen processing) before loading onto MHC class I molecules. The class I peptide/MHC complexes eventually exit the ER by association with B cell-associated protein Bap31.

Similarly to MHC class I molecules, MHC class II molecules are also synthesized in the ER. In addition to the polypeptide α and β chains, an invariant chain (Ii) is also produced within the ER, which associates with MHC class II molecules before

Published by Woodhead Publishing Limited, 2013

they reach the cell surface. Unlike MHC class I expression, which encompasses most cells, class II MHC expression is limited to specific antigen presenting cells (APCs) such as dendritic cells, endothelial cells, monocytes and B cells. They present exogenous peptide antigens to helper T cells through the TCR and CD4. Exogenous foreign antigen is processed through the MHC class II pathway. Antigen is internalized and degraded enzymatically in endosomes and lysosomes into peptide fragments. MHC class II molecules remain competent for peptide loading by binding fragments of Ii in the ER. These fragments remain bound while Ii targets the MHC class II molecule to a lysosomal-like compartment termed MHC class II compartment (MIIC). Within the MIIC, the Ii is removed from MHC class II molecules by the combined action of proteolytic enzymes and HLA-DM molecule, and the peptides are able to bind to the available peptide binding clefts of the class II molecules. Newly loaded class II molecules are subsequently translocated to the surface of APCs, where their interactions with helper T cells stimulate effector response by the production of cytokines.

1.4 Peptide binding

The binding of peptides to MHC class I molecules is a non-covalent interaction mediated by residues both in the peptides and in the clefts of the MHC molecules. Peptides of 7 to 14 residues bind to class I MHC molecules in an extended conformation. The amino acid residues of a peptide may contain side-chains that fit into polymorphic cavities (or "pockets") and bind to complementary amino acids in the MHC molecule. These residues are called anchor residues because they "anchor" the peptide firmly in the MHC binding cleft and contribute most of the favorable interactions

Published by Woodhead Publishing Limited, 2013

of the binding. There are typically two anchor residues, at the second (or fifth) and final peptide positions. The termini of the peptide are buried deep in the cleft and are bound by a set of conserved hydrogen bonds. Interestingly, this arrangement does not limit the length of the peptide. Longer peptides may zigzag or bulge to allow peptides of greater length to maintain the relative position of the termini, and peptides without the presence of canonical anchors have also been discovered to bind with high avidity to their respective MHC molecules. The peptide-binding cleft can be subdivided into six pockets (A to F). The polymorphic residues that line the peptide-binding cleft determine the individual specificity of peptide/MHC interaction.

Unlike class I, in which the allele-independent hydrogen bonding to the peptide is focused at the N- and C-termini, MHC class II molecules form hydrogen bonds along the entire length of the peptide with links to the atoms forming the main chain. The peptide-binding cleft of class II molecules can be subdivided into nine pockets (1 to 9). They possess an open binding cleft that does not constrain the length of the bound peptide, allowing the antigenic fragment to extend out of the binding cleft. Thus, each class II molecule can accommodate peptides with a spectrum of lengths ranging from nine to 30 amino acid residues.

1.5 Bibliography

1. Androlewicz, M.J., Ortmann, B., van Endert, P., Spies, T. and Cresswell, P. (1994) Characteristics of peptide and major histocompatibility complex class I/ ß2-microglobulin binding to the transporters associated with antigen processing (TAP1 and TAP2). *Proc. Natl. Acad. Sci. USA* **91**: 12 716–20.

Published by Woodhead Publishing Limited, 2013

2. Chen, W., Khilko, S., Fecondo, J., Margulies, D.H. and McCluskey, J. (1994) Determinant selection of major histocompatibility complex class I-restricted antigenic peptides is explained by class I-peptide affinity and is strongly influenced by nondominant anchor residues. *J. Exp. Med.* **180**: 1471–83.
3. Collins, E.J., Garboczi, D.N., Karpusas, M.N. and Wiley, D.C. (1995) The three-dimensional structure of a class I major histocompatibility complex molecule missing the alpha 3 domain of the heavy chain. *Proc. Natl. Acad. Sci. USA* **92**: 1218–21.
4. Cresswell, P. (1994) Assembly, transport, and function of MHC class II molecules. *Annu. Rev. Immunol.* **12**: 259–93.
5. Garrett, T.P.J., Saper, M.A., Bjorkman, P.J., Strominger, J.L. and Wiley, D.C. (1989) Specificity pockets for the side chains of peptide antigens in HLA-Aw68. *Nature* **342**: 692–6.
6. Gorer, P.A.J. (1937) *Pathol. Bacteriol.* **44**: 691.
7. Guo, H.C., Jardetzky, T.S., Garrett, T.P., Lane, W.S., Strominger, J.L. et al. (1992) Different length peptides bind to HLA-Aw68 similarly at their ends but bulge out in the middle. *Nature* **360**: 364–6.
8. Murthy, V.L. and Stern, L.J. (1997) The class II MHC protein HLA-DR1 in complex with an endogenous peptide: implications for the structural basis of the specificity of peptide binding. *Structure* **5**: 1385–96.
9. Jameson, S.C. and Bevan, M.J. (1992) Dissection of major histocompatibility complex (MHC) and T cell receptor contact residues in a Kb-restricted ovalbumin peptide and an assessment of the predictive power of MHC-binding motifs. *Eur. J. Immunol.* **22**: 2663–7.

Published by Woodhead Publishing Limited, 2013

10. Palmowski, M.J., Gileadi, U., Salio, M., Gallimore, A., Millrain, M., et al. (2006) Role of immunoproteasomes in cross-presentation. *J. Immunol.* **177**: 983–90.
11. Hanada, K., Yewdell, J.W. and Yang, J.C. (2004) Immune recognition of a human renal cancer antigen through post-translational protein splicing. *Nature* **427**: 252–6.
12. Yewdell, J.W., Reits, E. and Neefjes, J. (2003) Quantitating the MHC class I antigen processing pathway. *Nat. Rev. Immunol.* **3**: 952–61.
13. Momburg, F. and Hämmerling, G. (1998) Generation and TAP-mediated transport of peptides for major histocompatibility complex class I molecules. *Adv. Immunol.* **68**: 191–256.
14. Hammer, G.E., Gonzalez, F., Champsaur, M., Cado, D. and Shastri, N. (2005) The aminopeptidase ERAAP shapes the peptide repertoire displayed by major histocompatibility complex class I molecules. *Nat. Immunol.* **7**: 103–12.
15. Spiliotis, E.T., Manley, H., Osorio, M., Zuniga, M.C. and Edidin, M. (2000) Selective export of MHC class I molecules from the ER after their dissociation from TAP. *Immunity* **6**: 841–51.
16. Rudensky, A.Y., Maric, M., Eastman, S., Shoemaker, L., DeRoos, P.C., et al. (1994) Intracellular assembly and transport of endogenous peptide-MHC class II complexes. *Immunity* **1**: 585–94.
17. Peters, P.J., Raposo, G., Neefjes, J.J., Oorschot, V., Leijendekker, R.L., et al. (1995) Major histocompatibility complex class II compartments in human B lymphoblastoid cells are distinct from early endosomes. *J. Exp. Med.* **182**: 325–34.
18. Madden, D.R., Gorga, J.C., Strominger, J.L. and Wiley, D.C. (1992) The three-dimensional structure of

HLA-B27 at 2.1. Å resolution suggests a general mechanism for tight peptide binding to MHC. *Cell* 70: 1035–48.

19. Madden, D.R., Garboczi, D.N. and Wiley, D.C. (1993) The antigenic identity of peptide-MHC complexes: a comparison of the conformations of five viral peptides presented by HLA-A2. *Cell* 75: 693–708.
20. Stern, L.J. and Wiley, D.C. (1994) Antigenic peptide binding by class I and class II histocompatibility proteins. *Structure* 2: 245–51.

Published by Woodhead Publishing Limited, 2013

2

Immunoglobulins and B cell responses

DOI: 10.1533/9781908818416.13

Abstract: Immunoglobulins or antibodies are proteins that play a central role in humoral immune recognition by binding specifically to the antigens that induced their production. They are able to agglutinate insoluble antigens, rendering them ineffective, and induce the effector cells of the immune system. By coating pathogens, they prevent them from entering or damaging cells, stimulate their removal, and trigger their destruction by activating the complement system. Here, we describe the immunoglobulin classes in humans – IgA (found in body surfaces exposed to outside antigens), IgD (which may be involved in monitoring infection by respiratory bacteria), IgE (found in the lungs, skin and mucous membranes, and involved in allergic responses), IgG (the main antibody found in human serum, and the major antibody of the secondary response) and IgM (the first antibody to be produced in response to an infection) – and their respective roles in B cell-mediated immune responses. Their structures, properties, and functions are discussed.

Key words: immunoglobulin, antibody, isotype, humoral immune responses, B cell, B cell receptor.

Published by Woodhead Publishing Limited, 2013

2.1 Types of immunoglobulins

Immunoglobulins or antibodies are major players in B cell-mediated immune recognition that bind specifically to the antigens that induced their production. In humans, there are five distinct immunoglobulin (Ig) classes or isotypes: IgA, IgD, IgE, IgG and IgM. They differ in terms of their biological properties (i.e. amino acid composition, charge, size, and carbohydrate content), functional locations and their specificities for different antigens.

2.1.1 IgA

This subclass of antibody protects body surfaces that are exposed to outside foreign antigens. IgA is found in the gut, respiratory tract, and urogenital tract, as well as in colostrum, saliva, tears, and maternal milk. Two subclasses are found in humans – IgA_1 and IgA_2, with IgA_1 being predominantly (90%) expressed over IgA_2 (10%). Together, they constitute about 15% of the circulating antibodies.

2.1.2 IgD

This isotype is usually co-expressed with IgM. IgD can be found in the plasma membrane of circulating B cells but accounts for fewer than 1% of immunoglobulins present in the body. Circulating IgD may bind to basophils and orchestrate a surveillance system to monitor invasion by respiratory bacteria, and regulate antibody responses. However, the protein has a very short half-life as it is highly vulnerable to proteolytic attack.

Published by Woodhead Publishing Limited, 2013

2.1.3 IgE

IgE is a monomeric antibody that is found in the lungs, skin, and mucous membranes. This type of immunoglobulin is associated with allergic reactions, especially with type 1 hypersensitivity. It is present in extremely low levels (0.05%) in the serum and elicits an immune response by binding to Fc receptors on the surface of mast cells and basophils.

2.1.4 IgG

IgG is the smallest but most predominant immunoglobulin of serum (75%). It is also the major antibody of the secondary response, and its presence is usually associated with the maturation of antibody response. There are four subclasses in humans – IgG_1, IgG_2, IgG_3, and IgG_4. IgG plays an important role in fighting bacterial, viral, and fungal infections. It is the only type of antibody that can cross the human placenta to provide humoral immunity to the fetus in utero.

2.1.5 IgM

IgM is the largest immunoglobulin in the body, consisting of five monomer subunits linked by disulphide bridges. This type of antibody makes up 10% of circulating antibodies and is found in blood and lymph fluid. The protein is also the first immunoglobulin type to be produced in response to an infection.

2.2 Immunoglobulin structure

The basic functional unit of an immunoglobulin is a monomer of two light chains and two heavy chains linked by disulphide

Published by Woodhead Publishing Limited, 2013

bonds and non-covalent interactions (see Figure 2.1). In humans, there are two types of light chains – kappa (κ) and lambda (λ). An individual light chain has a molecular weight of 25 kDa and is approximately 211 to 217 amino acids long. Each light chain has two domains – a constant region termed C_L with amino acid sequences that are similar for the same isotype, and a variable region V_L with high variation in its primary sequence. The tertiary structure of C_L will determine whether the light chain is κ or λ, while the structure of V_L will determine its antigen specificity. The heavy chains adopt similar configurations to the light chains, with one domain that is similar for the same isotype (C_H), and one domain that is highly variable (V_H). There are five types of heavy chains – α, δ, ε, γ, and μ, each with a molecular weight of 50 to 75 kDa. The tertiary structure of the combined V_L and V_H domains defines the conformation of the antigen-binding site or paratope. As the two light and heavy chains are identical, each

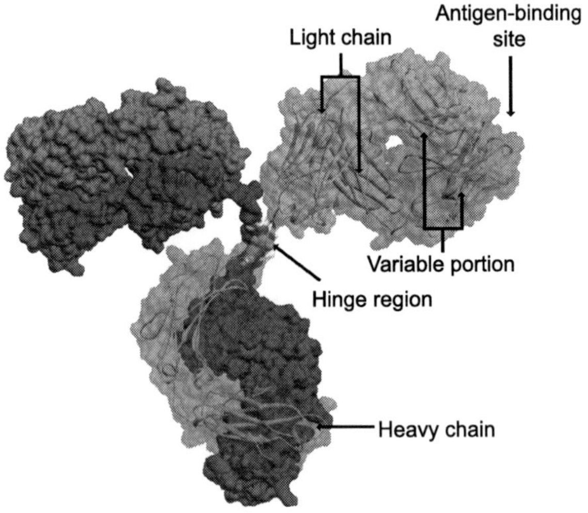

Figure 2.1 Schematic of an immunoglobulin molecule based on X-ray crystallographic structure

Published by Woodhead Publishing Limited, 2013

functional unit of an immunoglobulin contains two identical antigen-binding sites at the N-terminal of the molecule.

2.3 Immunoglobulin function

The main role of the immunoglobulin is to bind the antigen that triggered its formation. Each immunoglobulin has a different paratope, which allows it to bind different epitopes. Immunoglobulins contribute to immunity in three ways: they prevent pathogens from entering or damaging cells by binding to them; they stimulate removal of pathogens by phagocytosis and other effector mechanisms by coating the pathogen; and they trigger destruction of pathogens by activating the complement system.

2.3.1 Neutralization

For insoluble antigens such as animal cells, bacteria, or erythrocytes, cross-linking of adjacent antigens by a single immunoglobulin allows agglutination or clumping of pathogens to occur. The agglutinate helps to isolate the pathogen, prevents its dissemination and facilitates its removal through other immune-mediated functions. If the antigen is soluble, precipitation occurs for large complexes while small complexes remain in soluble form. By binding to functionally important residues on pathogens responsible for the establishment of infection, immunoglobulins serve to disrupt the viral infection process and neutralize their harmful effects.

2.3.2 Opsonization

Immunoglobulins function as flexible adapters mediating the adherence of antigens to effector cells of the immune system,

Published by Woodhead Publishing Limited, 2013

including dendritic cells, macrophages, monocytes, and myeloid cells. The Fc region of IgA, IgG and IgE can interact with the Fc receptors on the effector cells to induce cellular effector mechanisms, including phagocytosis, endocytosis, antibody-mediated cellular cytotoxicity, and the release of cytokines and cytotoxic molecules. The engagement of a single immunoglobulin with an effector cell is not sufficient to stimulate phagocytosis or other effector mechanisms. When an antigen is bound to many immunoglobulins, the collective interactions will then be enough to trigger the cell's effector function.

2.3.3 Complement activation

The complement system is a major effector mechanism of the immunoglobulins that mediates cell lysis and inflammatory reactions. It refers to a series of proteins, including serum proteins, serosal proteins, and cell membrane receptors, that circulate in the blood as inactive precursors. The complement cascade is activated when the Fc region of IgA, IgG, or IgM binds to an antigen. It comprises three complement pathways – the classical complement pathway, the alternate complement pathway, and the mannose-binding lectin pathway. The classical pathway is triggered by C1 proteins binding to antigen-bound IgG or IgM molecules. The alternate classical pathway is mediated by C3 proteins binding to microbes and immunoglobulin molecules. Compared with the classical pathway, it has a faster response time, as it does not require a specific immunoglobulin to commence. The lectin pathway is activated when microbial carbohydrates interact with mannan-binding lectin (MBL) in the plasma and tissue fluids. It is similar to the alternate classical pathway in that it is not immunoglobulin dependent.

Published by Woodhead Publishing Limited, 2013

2.4 Antigen binding

The interactions of antigens with immunoglobulins involve binding to antigenic determinants or epitopes on the surface of antigen molecules. The immunoglobulin binding site is predominantly hydrophobic, formed by three hypervariable loops of diverse length and amino acid composition. About 10% of B cell epitopes are contiguous, consisting of a linear stretch of amino acids along the polypeptide chain. Most epitopes, though, are non-contiguous or conformational in nature, whereby distantly separated residues of the polypeptide chain are brought into spatial proximity by protein folding. The primary sequences of B cell epitopes are poorly conserved and difficult to characterize. It is known that not all residues within an epitope are functionally important for binding. Antibodies with dissimilar binding site structures may exhibit similar specificities for common epitopes, and the specificity could be reduced or eliminated by single-site amino acid substitution.

2.5 Bibliography

1. Alzari, P.M., Lascombe, M.–B. and Poljak, R.J. (1988) Three-dimensional structure of antibodies. *Annu. Rev. Immunol.* **6**: 555–80.
2. Balkwill, F.R. and Burke, F. (1989) The cytokine network. *Immunol. Today* **10**: 299–304.
3. Butcher, E.C. (1990) Cellular and molecular mechanisms that direct leukocyte traffic. *Am. J. Pathol.* **136**: 1–11.
4. Chen, K., Xu, W., Wilson, M., He, B., Miller, N.W., et al. (2009) Immunoglobulin D enhances immune surveillance by activating antimicrobial,

Published by Woodhead Publishing Limited, 2013

pro-inflammatory and B cell-stimulating programs in basophils. *Nat. Immunol.* **10**: 889–98.

5. Wiersma, E.J., Collins, C., Fazel, S. and Shulman, M.J. (1998) Structural and functional analysis of J chain-deficient IgM. *J. Immunol.* **160**: 5979–89.
6. Gould, H.J., Sutton, B.J., Beavil, A.J., McCloskey, N., Coker, H.A., et al. (2003) The biology of IgE and the basis of allergic disease. *Annu. Rev. Immunol.* **21**: 579–628.
7. Ohta, Y. and Flajnik, M. (2006) IgD, like IgM, is a primordial immunoglobulin class perpetuated in most jawed vertebrates. *Proc. Natl. Acad. Sci. USA* **103**: 10 723–8.
8. Simell, B., Kilpi, T. and Käyhty, H. (2006) Subclass distribution of natural salivary IgA antibodies against pneumococcal capsular polysaccharide of type 14 and pneumococcal surface adhesin A (PsaA) in children. *Clin. Exp. Immunol.* **143**: 543–9.
9. Nair, D.T., Singh, K., Sahu, N., Rao, K.V. and Salunke, D.M. (2000) Crystal structure of an antibody bound to an immunodominant peptide epitope: novel features in peptide-antibody recognition. *J. Immunol.* **165**: 6949–55.
10. Poljak, R.J. (1991) Structure of antibodies and their complexes with antigens. *Mol. Immunol.* **28**: 1341–5.
11. Barlow, D.J., Edwards, M.S. and Thornton, J.M. (1986) Continuous and discontinuous protein antigenic determinants. *Nature* **322**: 747–8.
12. Helm, R.M., Cockrell, G., Connaughton, C., West, C.M., Herman, E., et al. (2000) Mutational analysis of the IgE-binding epitopes of P34/Gly m Bd30 K. *J. Allergy Clin. Immunol.* **105**: 378–84.
13. Nair, D.T., Singh, K., Siddigui, Z., Nayak, B.P., Rao, K.V., et al. (2002) Epitope recognition by diverse antibodies suggests conformational convergence in an antibody response. *J. Immunol.* **168**: 2371–82.

Published by Woodhead Publishing Limited, 2013

3

Scientific publications and databases

DOI: 10.1533/9781908818416.21

Abstract: Scientific literature in the form of formal academic publications, scholarly books, book chapters, dissertations, and meeting presentations is the primary source of information for the scientific community. Today, most of this information is available electronically and can be found on the Web. Many articles are now open access, so that the scientific community can read the full text instantly, and the use of hyperlinks has fundamentally changed the structure and delivery of information. In this chapter, we survey the digital libraries that are available to the biomedical community, including tools for retrieving biomedical literature (such as the search engines PubMed and Google Scholar), general databases for storing information on genes and proteins, and immunological databases for research into autoimmune disorders, infectious diseases, cancer, immunotherapy, and immunoprophylaxis.

Key words: biological databases, immunological databases, scientific publications, molecular biology databases, search engines.

Published by Woodhead Publishing Limited, 2013

3.1 Bibliographical information

The history of scientific journals can be traced back to 1665, when the French *Journal des sçavans* and the English *Philosophical Transactions of the Royal Society* first began systematically publishing research results. Academic papers are assessed by scientific peers to ensure that the results are sound and significant. Today, formal academic publications continue to serve as the primary medium for the dissemination of scientific results. In addition, scholarly books, book chapters, dissertations, and meeting presentations all contribute to the diverse formats of scientific publications that we see today.

The emergence of the Internet heralded a new dawn in the way regular scientific literature is being distributed. In pre-Internet times, articles existed primarily in printed form, and scientists visited the library regularly to perform fact findings and read up on the latest discoveries and trends. Today, most journals and books are available electronically and can be found on the Web. The PubMed database, from the US National Library of Medicine, currently indexes more than 21 million citations for biomedical literature from MEDLINE, life science journals, and online books published from 1966 until the present. Many articles are now open access, so the scientific community will be able to read the full text instantly. The proliferation of digital libraries has changed the fundamental way in which information can be accessed:

- Scientific literature is no longer localized within the constraints of paper copies at one or more physical locations, and is available anywhere at any time with Internet access.
- Information flow is no longer within the confines of a single dimension, where readers follow the content of a

Published by Woodhead Publishing Limited, 2013

book on a line-by-line basis. Hyperlinks fundamentally change how information is being delivered. Internal links point users to other sections of the main text, or to an image, sound, or movie within the current document. External links point readers to other sources containing related or supplementary information. Selecting the hyperlinks from those sources will point you to further information, and so on and so forth.

- Search engines now play an essential role in information retrieval. Full text search is the simplest and most commonly used method for locating information in relevant web sites, including those published in scientific literature. More sophisticated search engines allow synonym, wildcard or fuzzy searches using the search word, or matched pattern in the string.

3.2 Searching the literature

The Medical Literature Analysis and Retrieval System Online (MEDLINE) is the bibliographic database of the US National Library of Medicine (NLM), containing journal citations and abstracts for biomedical literature from all around the world. The database currently houses over 21 million records from ~5000 publications starting from 1950. MEDLINE uses Medical Subject Headings (MeSH) for information retrieval, and is searchable using NLM's National Center for Biotechnology Information (NCBI)'s PubMed (see Figure 3.1).

PubMed was started in January 1996 by NCBI as an experimental search system with full access to MEDLINE. In April 1997, the word "experimental" was dropped from the web site. PubMed searches typically exceeded 50 million per month in 2009. The system allows:

Published by Woodhead Publishing Limited, 2013

- Simple text searches and automatic term mapping using a MeSH table, a Journals translation table, a Full Author translation table, Author index, the Full Investigator translation table, and an Investigator index. When a match is found for a term or phrase in a translation table, the mapping process is complete and does not continue on to the next translation table.
- Advanced text searches using a combination of user-defined field names, Boolean operators, search tags, and automatic term mapping.

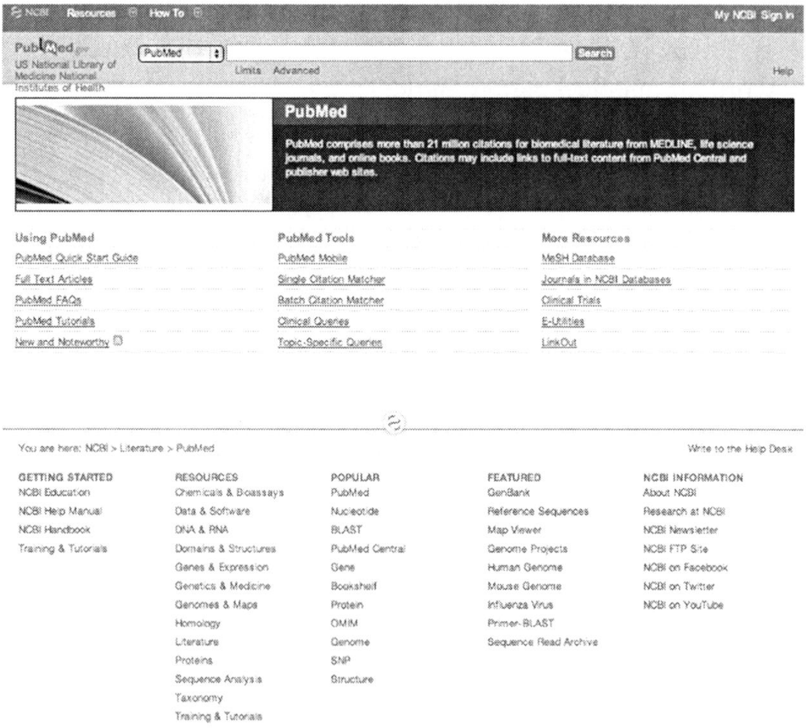

Figure 3.1 PubMed homepage containing a search bar at the top of the site and hyperlinks to various tools and resources at the bottom

Published by Woodhead Publishing Limited, 2013

In November 2004, Google Inc. launched Google Scholar, a specialized search engine that covers academic publications, including peer-reviewed papers, technical reports, preprints, theses, books, abstracts, and selected web pages that are deemed by the company to be "scholarly" in nature. Similar to the Google search engine, it is fast and easy to use. The system retrieves relevant documents based on keyword searches, but lacks advanced features such as MeSH mapping, nested Boolean searching, or publication type limits.

3.3 General databases containing information on genes and proteins

Currently, a great variety of databases on different aspects of molecular biology and small molecules are available. The yearly Nucleic Acids Research (NAR) Molecular Biology Database Collection (*http://www3.oup.co.uk/nar/database/c/*) catalogues new and updated molecular biology databases that are freely available on the web. More than 1300 data sources have been published in 18 editions. Most of these databases focus on a specific topic. Each may have a different scope, but most contain a unifying theme.

3.3.1 GenBank/EMBL-Bank/DDBJ

The international collaborative GenBank, DNA Data Bank of Japan (DDBJ) and European Molecular Biology Laboratory (EMBL) Nucleotide Sequence Database serve as worldwide repositories for all publicly available nucleotide sequences.

GenBank, developed and maintained by the US National Institute of Health (NIH)'s NCBI, is accessible through the NCBI Entrez retrieval system. The database primarily contains

Published by Woodhead Publishing Limited, 2013

sequence data collected from direct submission of authors, bulk submission of expressed sequence tag (EST), genome survey sequence (GSS), whole genome shotgun (WGS), high-throughput data from sequencing centers, and sequence information from patents issued by the US Office of Patents and Trademarks. Nucleotide sequences may be submitted to GenBank via the BankIt web-based sequence submission form, or the Sequin standalone submission program available at its website. The database is released bimonthly, and is available at *http://www.ncbi.nlm.nih.gov/genbank/*.

The EMBL Nucleotide Sequence Database, otherwise known as EMBL-Bank, is part of the European Nucleotide Archive (ENA) aimed at constructing a comprehensive catalog of the world's nucleotide sequencing information. Maintained by the European Bioinformatics Institute (EBI), the database represents Europe's primary nucleotide sequence resource. New versions of EMBL-Bank are released on a quarterly basis and can be accessed via ftp and several web interfaces. The nucleotide sequence database is divided into 17 divisions, with each record being assigned to a specific division based on the nature of the data – bacteriophage, ESTs, fungi, high-throughput genome, genome survey sequences, humans, invertebrates, organelles, other mammals, other vertebrates, plants, prokaryotes, rodents, sequence-tagged sites (STSs), synthetic, unclassified, and viruses. EMBL-Bank is available at *http://www.ebi.ac.uk/embl/*.

DDBJ is developed by the Center for Information Biology and DDBJ (CIB-DDBJ) of the National Institute of Genetics (NIG) of Japan, with funding support by the Japanese Ministry of Education, Culture, Sports, Science and Technology (MEXT). It was established in 1986 through collaboration with the EBI in Europe and NCBI in USA. DDBJ serves as the only nucleotide sequence archive database in Asia. The database mainly collects original DNA data

Published by Woodhead Publishing Limited, 2013

from Japanese researchers, with the remainder from China, Korea, Taiwan, and other countries. These sequences are then annotated and subsequently disseminated to the public. DDBJ is freely accessible at *http://www.ddbj.nig.ac.jp*.

GenBank, EMBL-Bank, and DDBJ each collect a portion of the total nucleotide sequence data worldwide, and synchronize their records on a daily basis within the framework of the International Nucleotide Sequence Database Collaboration (INSDC). As of September 2012, the databases contained over 126 billion nucleotide bases in more than 135 million reported sequences.

3.3.2 UniProt

The UniProt database, jointly developed by the European Bioinformatics Institute (EBI), the Swiss Institute of Bioinformatics (SIB), and the Protein Information Resource (PIR), is widely considered as the central resource for protein sequence and functional information (see Figure 3.2). Presently, UniProt comprises four components:

1. The UniProt Knowledgebase (UniProtKB) serves as a repository for curated protein information, including sequence, function, classification, and cross-references to key biological databases. UniProtKB is divided into two sections: a) UniProtKB/Swiss-Prot, which is manually annotated and reviewed by experts, and b) UniProt/TrEMBL (Translated EMBL), which is a computer-annotated protein sequence database supplement of Swiss-Prot that includes all translation of EMBL nucleotide sequences not available in the database.
2. The UniProt Reference Clusters (UniRef) databases contain clustered sets of sequences from the UniProtKB and selected UniProt Archive records. There are three

Published by Woodhead Publishing Limited, 2013

versions of UniRef: UniRef100, UniRef90, and UniRef50, representing the resolutions of non-redundant sequences at sequence identity levels of at least 100%, 90%, and 50%, respectively.

3. The UniProt Archive (UniParc) is a comprehensive and non-redundant database used to keep track of protein sequences from major public databases including UniProt/Swiss-Prot, UniProtKB/TrEMBL, PIR-PSD, EMBL, EMBL WGS, Ensembl, IPI, PDB, PIR-PSD, RefSeq, FlyBase, WormBase, H-Invitational Database, TROME database, European Patent Office proteins, United States Patent and Trademark Office proteins (USPTO), and Japan Patent Office proteins.
4. The UniProt Metagenomic and Environmental Sequences (UniMES) database is a repository containing metagenomic and environmental data.

3.3.3 PDB

Protein Data Bank (PDB) is the single worldwide archive of structural data of biological macromolecules. It includes data obtained by X-ray crystallography and nuclear magnetic resonance (NMR) spectrometry submitted by biologists and biochemists from all over the world. Presently, PDB is under the purview of the Worldwide Protein Data Bank (wwPDB), a network of four organizations – Research Collaboratory for Structural Bioinformatics (RCSB) PDB (USA), PDB in Europe (PDBe) (Europe), PDB Japan (PDBj) (Japan), and the Biological Magnetic Resonance Data Bank (BMRB) (USA) – whose mission is to "maintain a single Protein Data Bank Archive of macromolecular structural data that is freely and publicly available to the global community." Currently, more than 83 900 biological macromolecular structures have been

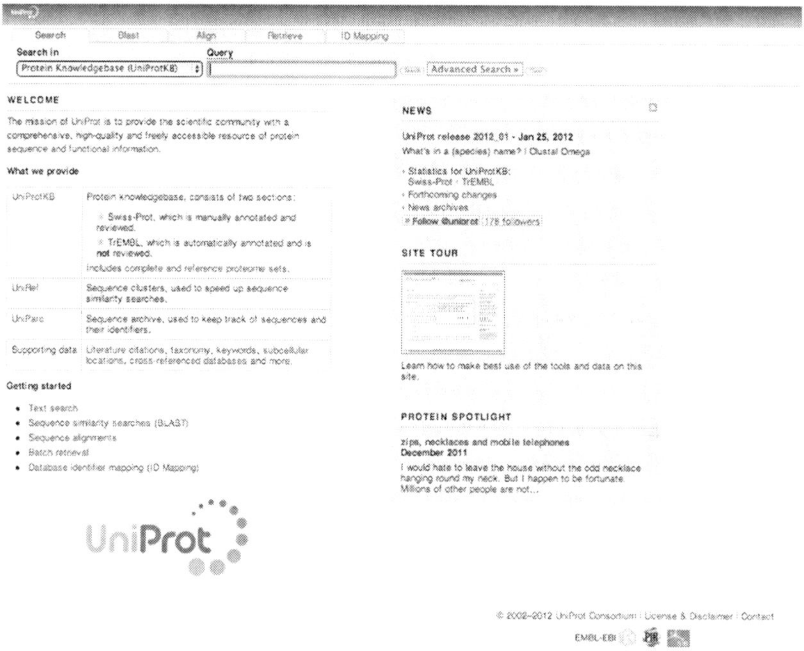

Figure 3.2 UniProt homepage with a search bar that allows users to perform queries on i) core data such as Protein Knowledgebase (UniProtKB), Sequence Clusters (UniRef), and Sequence Archive (UniParc), ii) supporting data such as literature citations, taxonomy, keywords, subcellular locations, and cross-referenced databases, and iii) other information including news, documents, and user manual

deposited in PDB. The database is freely accessible at *http://www.rcsb.org/*.

3.4 Immunological databases

Immunological databases and web services have been proliferating over the past decade. More than 30

Published by Woodhead Publishing Limited, 2013

immunological databases are now available in the NAR Molecular Biology Database Collection. Immune epitope databases are useful for MHC, T cell receptor (TR) and Ig binding analysis, with direct applications in component vaccine design and analysis of host–pathogen interactions. Immune sequence databases are valuable for research in autoimmune disorders, infectious diseases, cancer, immunotherapy, and immunoprophylaxis. The most important databases are described below.

3.4.1 IEDB

The Immune Epitope Database (IEDB; *http://www.iedb.org*; see Figure 3.3), funded by the National Institute of Allergy and Infectious Diseases (NIAID), is presently considered as a central resource for experimentally characterized B and T cell epitopes, as well as MHC ligand information for humans, non-human primates, rodents, pigs, cats, and other animal

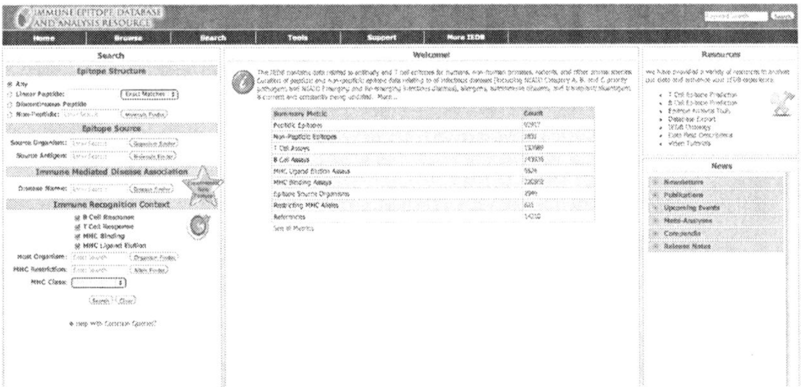

Figure 3.3 IEDB homepage. Users can perform queries based on the epitope structure, epitope source, immune-mediated disease association, and immune recognition context

Published by Woodhead Publishing Limited, 2013

species. Development of the database began in 2004 at the La Jolla Institute for Allergy and Immunology, with the aim of cataloging all experimentally derived information on immune epitopes from the literature and from direct submission by laboratories generating the data. Records of epitopes derived from the literature are linked to their reference sources, and include information such as authors, article title, journal name, and abstract. The database includes peptidic and non-peptidic epitope data relating to NIAID Category A, B and C priority pathogens and NIAID emerging and re-emerging infectious diseases, other infectious diseases, allergens, and autoantigens. IEDB now contains information on around 93 000 peptidic epitopes and 1800 non-peptidic epitopes from over 2900 source organisms, representing ~99% of all publicly available information on peptide epitopes from infectious agents and ~93% of epitopes from allergens.

3.4.2 SYFPEITHI

SYFPEITHI (*http://www.syfpeithi.de/*), developed by Hans-Georg Rammensee's group at the Department of Immunology, Tübingen, in 1999, is the first publicly available database for MHC ligands and peptide motifs (see Figure 3.4). The name SYFPEITHI was selected by the group to acknowledge the first MHC-eluted peptide that was directly sequenced. Presently, the database contains more than 7000 T cell epitopes, MHC ligands, and MHC-peptide motifs of humans and other species, including apes, cattle, chickens, and mice.

3.4.3 AntiJen

AntiJen (*http://www.ddg-pharmfac.net/antijen/*), developed by Darren Flower's group at the Edward Jenner Institute for

Published by Woodhead Publishing Limited, 2013

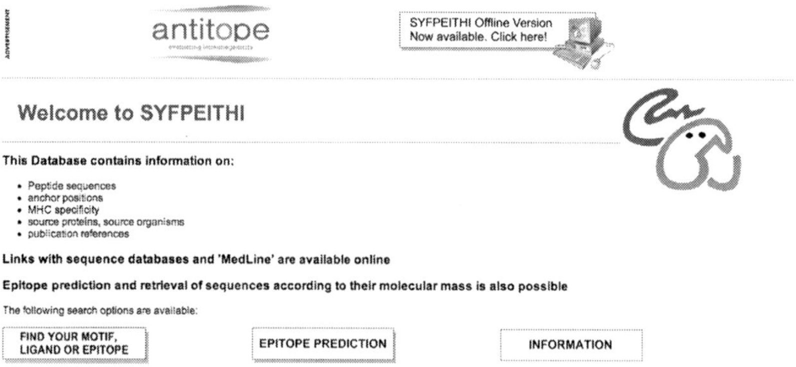

Figure 3.4 SYFPEITHI homepage, with links to tools for motif, ligand, and epitope search and prediction

Vaccine Research, is a repository containing quantitative binding data for MHC ligands, TR/peptide/MHC complexes, T cell epitopes, TAP, B cell epitopes and general immunological protein–protein interactions. The database is one of the largest immune epitope databases presently available, with over 24 000 records, and includes quantitative specificity data from position-specific peptide libraries and biophysical data, in the form of diffusion coefficients and cell surface copy numbers, on MHCs and other immunological molecules.

3.4.4 MHCBN

MHCBN (*http://www.imtech.res.in/raghava/mhcbn/*) is another major database containing information on peptides binding to MHC and TAP molecules. Developed by Gagendra Raghava's group at the Institute of Microbial Technology in India, the fourth version of MHCBN comprises over 25 800 experimentally validated peptide sequences from published

Published by Woodhead Publishing Limited, 2013

literature and existing publicly available immunological databases.

3.4.5 MPID-T

The MHC–peptide interaction database-TR (MPID-T) (see Figure 3.5), developed by Shoba Ranganathan's group first at the National University of Singapore in 2006 and then at the Macquarie University in 2011, is a repository for sequence–structure–function information on TR/peptide/MHC interactions. TR/peptide/MHC and peptide/MHC interaction information that is stored in MPID-T includes

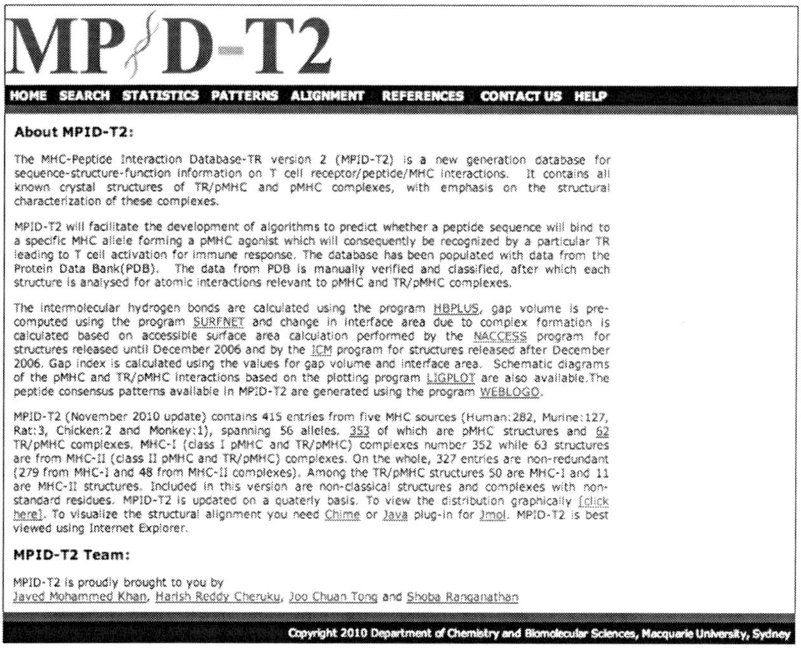

Figure 3.5 MPID-T homepage. The database contains sequence–structure–function information on 415 T cell receptor/peptide/MHC interactions

solvent accessibility, hydrogen bonds, non-hydrogen bonds, gap volume, gap index, interface area, and contact residues. In September 2012, the database contains 415 manually curated entries from human (282), murine (127), rat (3), chicken (2) and monkey (1) extracted from the PDB, of which 353 are peptide/MHC structures and 62 are TR/ peptide/MHC complexes. MHC class I complexes number 352 while 63 structures are from MHC class II complexes. On the whole, 327 entries are non-redundant (MHC class I: 279, MHC class II: 48). The present database also includes non-classical structures and complexes with non-standard residues. MPID-T is available at *http://biolinfo.org/mpid-t2/*.

3.4.6 BEID

The B cell epitope interaction database (BEID; *http://datam.i2r.a-star.edu.sg/BEID*), developed by Joo Chuan Tong's group at the Institute for Infocomm Research in Singapore, is a public database describing sequence–structure–function information on Ig–antigen interactions. In September 2012, the database contains 164 entries of antigen, 126 entries of Ig, and 189 complex entries of Ig–antigen complexes extracted from the PDB. Each record is manually verified, classified, and analyzed for atomic interactions between antigens and the corresponding bound Ig molecules. Ig–antigen interaction information that is stored in BEID includes solvent accessibility, hydrogen bonds, non-hydrogen bonds, gap volume, gap index, interface area, and contact residues.

3.4.7 CED

The Conformational Epitope Database (CED; *http://immunet.cn/ced/*) is a boutique database that stores manually

Published by Woodhead Publishing Limited, 2013

curated information on conformational B cell epitopes and related information including the composition and location of the epitope, the immunological property of the epitope, the source antigen, and the corresponding bound Ig molecules. As of September 2012, CED contains 225 records of epitopes from protein antigens (213), nucleic acids (6), glycans (5), and lipids (1), derived from humans (109), viruses (54), bacteria (22), invertebrates (7), plants (2), and other sources (2).

3.4.8 IMGT

The international ImMunoGeneTics information system® or IMGT® is a useful repository for Ig, TR, MHC, and related proteins of the immune system of humans and other vertebrates. IMGT is available at *http://imgt.org* (see Figure 3.6). It contains seven databases:

- IMGT/LIGM-DB is the comprehensive IMGT database for fully annotated nucleotide sequences of Ig and TR from human and other vertebrate species. In September 2012, IMGT/LIGM-DB contains 164 013 Ig and TR sequences from humans and 280 vertebrate species.
- IMGT/MH-DB is a specialist database for HLA sequences. It includes all the official sequences for the WHO Nomenclature Committee For Factors of the HLA System. In September 2012, the database contains sequences of 6292 HLA class I alleles, 1724 HLA class II alleles, 143 non-HLA alleles and 16 confidential alleles.
- IMGT/GENE-DB is a comprehensive database for Ig and TR genomic data. In September 2012, the database contains 2895 genes and 4141 alleles of human, mouse, rat and rabbit Ig and TR genes.

Published by Woodhead Publishing Limited, 2013

- IMGT/PRIMER-DB is the IMGT oligonucleotide (primer) database for Ig and TR. Ig and TR primers are used in combinatorial library design, antibody single chain Fragment variable (scFv), phage display, and microarray technologies. In September 2012, the database contains 1864 primer records of Ig and TR from 11 species.
- IMGT/CLL-DB is a specialist database that contains primary Ig sequences associated with biological and

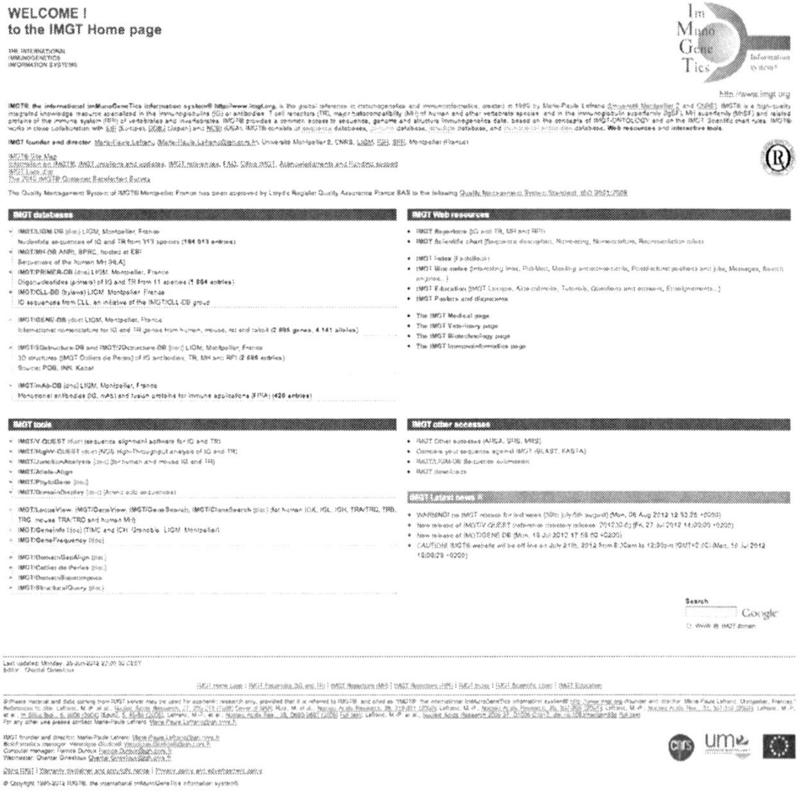

Figure 3.6 IMGT homepage, with links to wide array of information and resources in immunogenetics and immunoinformatics

Published by Woodhead Publishing Limited, 2013

clinical data for patients with chronic lymphocytic leukemia (CLL) attending academic institutions. Access to the database is currently restricted to members of the IMGT/CLL-DB group.

- IMGT/3Dstructure-DB is the IMGT annotated structural database for Ig, TR, MHC, and the related proteins of the immune system (RPI) belonging to the Ig superfamily and to the MHC superfamily. In September 2012, the database contains 2686 records of Ig, TR, MHC, and RPI proteins with known 3D structures.
- IMGT/mAb-DB is the IMGT monoclonal antibodies database. In September 2012, the database contains 420 records of monoclonal antibodies with clinical indications and fusion proteins for immune applications.

3.4.9 IPD

The Immuno Polymorphism Database (IPD; *http://www.ebi.ac.uk/ipd/*; see Figure 3.7) was developed in 2003 as a collaborative project between the HLA Informatics Group of the Anthony Nolan Research Institute and the European Bioinformatics Institute (EBI) to study polymorphism in genes of the immune system. It is made up of four specialist databases:

- IPD-KIR contains the allelic sequences of more than 600 killer-cell immunoglobulin-like receptors;
- IPD-MHC details the MHC sequences of a number of different species, including canines, cattle, chickens, felines, fish, horses, non-human primates, pinnipeds, prosimians, rats, sheep, and swine;
- IPD-HPA stores data which define the human platelet antigens;

Published by Woodhead Publishing Limited, 2013

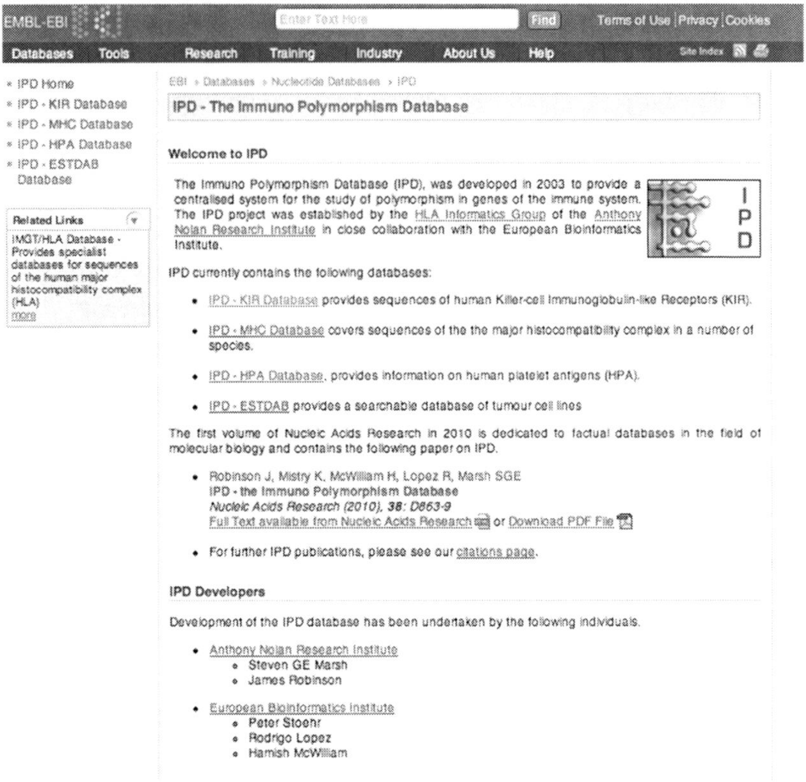

Figure 3.7 IPD homepage, with links to four specialist immunogenetic databases

- IPD-ESTAB provides access to the European Searchable Tumour Cell-Line Database (ESTDAB), a cell bank of immunologically characterized melanoma cell lines.

3.4.10 *The HIV Molecular Immunology Database*

The HIV Molecular Immunology Database, developed by the Los Alamos National Laboratory and funded by the Division of AIDS of the NIAID, is an annotated repository of

Published by Woodhead Publishing Limited, 2013

HIV-1 cytotoxic and helper T cell epitopes and Ig binding sites. As of September 2012, the database contains information on 905 HIV-1 cytotoxic T cell epitopes, 1023 HIV-1 helper T cell epitopes, and 1448 Ig binding sites. The HIV Molecular Immunology Database is publicly available at *http://www.hiv.lanl.gov/content/immunology/*.

3.5 Small molecule databases

3.5.1 ACD

The Accelrys Available Chemicals Directory (ACD; *http://accelrys.com/products/databases/sourcing/available-chemicals-directory.html*) is a commercial database for chemical sourcing in pharmaceutical, biotechnology, chemical, and agrochemical companies. As of September 2012, the database contains information on over 7 million unique chemicals, including 3D models, over 13 million products and over 35 million packages from around 900 suppliers.

3.5.2 ChemDB

ChemDB (*http://cdb.ics.uci.edu/*) is a public repository of small molecules on the Web. As of September 2012, the database contains ~5 million commercially available compounds for use as synthetic building blocks, as probes in systems biology and as leads for drug discovery. The chemical data are available in diverse formats including SMILES strings, 2D graphs of atoms and bonds, 3D atom coordinates, and fingerprints.

3.5.3 DrugBank

DrugBank (*http://www.drugbank.ca/*) is a richly annotated database containing data on the nomenclature, ontology,

Published by Woodhead Publishing Limited, 2013

chemistry, structure, function, action, pharmacology, pharmacokinetics, metabolism, and pharmaceutical properties of both small molecule and large molecule drugs. As of September 2012, the database stores information on 6711 drugs, including 1447 FDA-approved small molecule drugs, 131 FDA-approved biotech drugs, 85 nutraceuticals and 5080 experimental drugs. These entries are linked to 4227 non-redundant protein sequences that function as either drug targets, enzymes, transporters, or carriers.

3.5.4 NCI Open Database

The National Cancer Institute (NCI) Open Database (*http://cactus.nci.nih.gov/download/nci/*) is a freely accessible small molecule database containing compounds from both organic synthesis and natural source extracts. As of September 2012, a total of 266 151 structures are available in the database.

3.5.5 PubChem

PubChem (*http://pubchem.ncbi.nlm.nih.gov/*), under the umbrella of NIH Molecular Library Roadmap Initiative (*http://nihroadmap.nih.gov/*), is a small molecule database containing information on more than 40 million compounds and 19 million unique structures (see Figure 3.8). The database is organized as three linked components: PubChem BioAssay, PubChem Compound, and PubChem Substance. A tool is also available that allows chemical structure similarity search.

3.5.6 WOMBAT

THE World of Molecular BioAcTivity (WOMBAT), indexed by Sunset Molecular Discovery LLC (*http://www.*

Published by Woodhead Publishing Limited, 2013

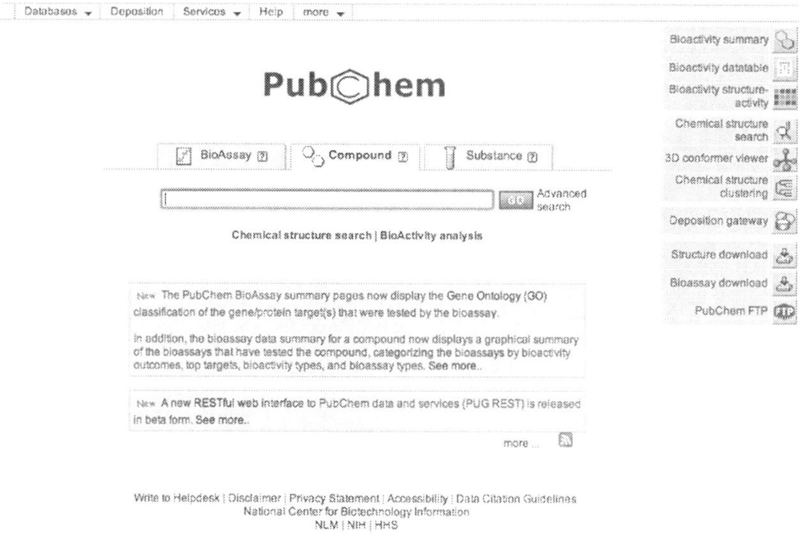

Figure 3.8 PubChem homepage, with tools for chemical structure similarity search and bioactivity analysis

sunsetmolecular.com/), is a commercial database for small molecules and their associated biological activities. The database is updated twice a year. As of September 2012, WOMBAT contains 331 872 entries representing 1966 unique targets from 15 320 medicinal chemistry journal papers between 1975 and 2009.

3.5.7 ZINC

ZINC (*http://zinc.docking.org/*; see Figure 3.9), maintained by Brian Shoichet's lab at the University of California, San Francisco, is a major small molecule database containing over 21 million purchasable compounds in ready-to-dock, three-dimensional formats. Most of the compounds have been corrected for protonation states and have the charges

Published by Woodhead Publishing Limited, 2013

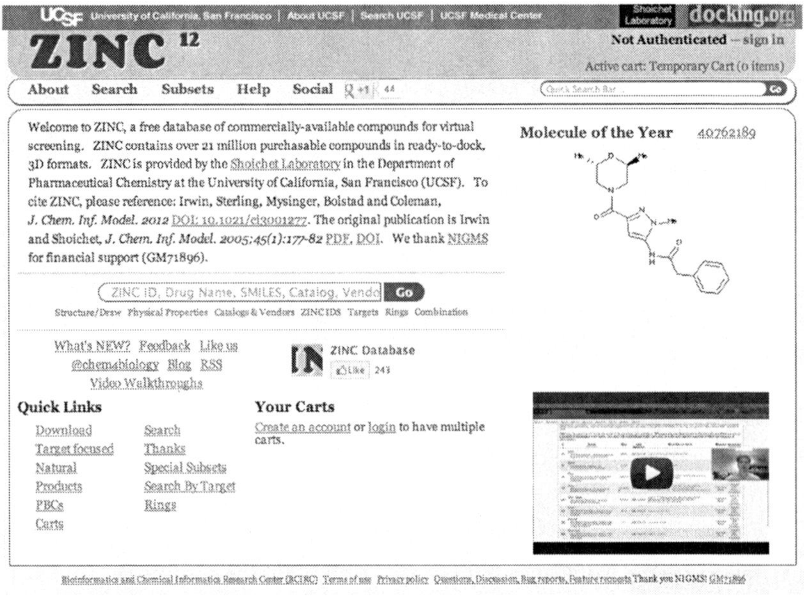

Figure 3.9 ZINC homepage, developed by the Shoichet Laboratory in the Department of Pharmaceutical Chemistry at the University of California, San Francisco

incorporated into the file. Other important properties, such as MW, calculated logP, and rotatable bonds, and multiple conformations are annotated into these files. In addition, the database also provides information on the vendors for the compounds, facilitating the purchase of compounds after the biological screens.

3.6 Bibliography

1. Jónsdóttir, S.O., Jørgensen, F.S. and Brunak, S. (2005) Prediction methods and databases within chemoinformatics: emphasis on drugs and drug candidates. *Bioinformatics* **21**: 2145–60.

2. Benson, D.A., Karsch-Mizrarchi, I., Lipman, D.J., Ostell, J. and Wheeler, D.L. (2006) GenBank. *Nucleic Acids Res.* 34: D16–20.
3. Tateno, Y., Imanishi, T., Miyazaki, S., Fukami-Kobayashi, K., Saitou, N., et al. (2002) DNA Data Bank of Japan (DDBJ) for genome scale research in life science. *Nucleic Acids Res.* 30: 27–30.
4. Kanz, C., Aldebert, P., Althorpe, N., Baker, W., Bates, K., et al. (2005) The EMBL nucleotide sequence database. *Nucleic Acids Res.* 33: D29–33.
5. O'Donovan, C., Martin, M.J., Gattiker, A., Gasteiger, E., Bairoch, A., et al. (2002) High-quality protein knowledge resource: SWISS-PROT and TrEMBL. *Brief. Bioinform.* 3: 275–84.
6. Wu, C.H., Huang, H., Arminski, L., Castro-Alvear, J., Chen, Y., et al. (2002) The protein information resource: an integrated public resource of functional annotation of proteins. *Nucleic Acids Res.* 30: 35–7.
7. Westbrook, J., Feng, Z., Jain, S., Bhat, T.N., Thanki, N., et al. (2002) The protein data bank: unifying the archive. *Nucleic Acids Res.* 30: 245–8.
8. Leinonen, R., Akhtar, R., Birney, E., Bower, L., Cerdeno-Tárraga, A., et al. (2011) The European nucleotide archive. *Nucleic Acids Res.* 39: D28–31.
9. Karsch-Mizrachi, I., Nakamura, Y. and Cochrane, G.; on behalf of the International Nucleotide Sequence Database Collaboration. (2012) The international nucleotide sequence database collaboration. *Nucleic Acids Res.* 40: D33–7.
10. Tateno, Y., Imanishi, T., Miyazaki, S., Fukami-Kobayashi, K., Saitou, N., et al. (2002) DNA Data Bank of Japan (DDBJ) for genome scale research in life science. *Nucleic Acids Res.* 30: 27–30.

Published by Woodhead Publishing Limited, 2013

11. Ponomarenko, J., Papangelopoulos, N., Zajonc, D.M., Peters, B., Sette, A., et al. (2011) IEDB-3D: structural data within the immune epitope database. *Nucleic Acids Res.* **39**: D1164–70.
12. Rammensee, H.G., Friede, T. and Stevanoviíc, S. (1995) MHC ligands and peptide motifs: first listing. *Immunogenetics* **41**: 178–228.
13. Rammensee, H.G., Bachmann, J., Emmerich, N.P., Bachor, O.A. and Stevanoviíc, S. (1999) *Immunogenetics* **50**: 213–19.
14. Tong, J.C., Song, C.M., Tan, P.T.J., Ren, E.C. and Sinha, A.A. (2008) BEID: database for sequence-structure-function information on antigen-antibody interactions. *Bioinformation* **3**: 58–60.
15. Lefranc, M.-P., Giudicelli, V., Kaas, Q., Duprat, E., Jabado-Michaloud, J., et al. (2005) IMGT, the international ImMunoGeneTics information system®. *Nucleic Acids Res.* **33**: D593–D597.
16. Lefranc, M.-P., Clément, O., Kaas, Q., Duprat, E., Chastellan, P., et al. (2005) IMGT-Choreography for Immunogenetics and Immunoinformatics. *In Silico Biol.* **5**: 45–60.
17. Giudicelli, V. and Lefranc, M.-P. (1999) Ontology for immunogenetics: the IMGT-ONTOLOGY. *Bioinformatics* **15**: 1047–54.
18. Duroux, P., Kaas, Q., Brochet, X., Lane, J., Ginestoux, C., et al. (2008) IMGT-Kaleidoscope, the formal IMGT-ONTOLOGY paradigm. *Biochimie* **90**: 570–83.
19. Khan, J.M., Cheruku, H.R., Tong, J.C. and Ranganathan, S. (2011) MPID-T2: a database for sequence-structure-function analyses of pMHC and TR/pMHC structures. *Bioinformatics* **27**: 1192–3.
20. Tong, J.C., Kong, L., Tan, T.W. and Ranganathan, S. (2006) MPID-T: database for sequence-structure-

function information on T-cell receptor/peptide/MHC interactions. *Appl. Bioinformatics* 5: 111–14.
21. Govindarajan, K.R., Kangueane, P., Tan, T.W. and Ranganathan, S. (2003) MPID: MHC-peptide interaction database for sequence-structure-function information on peptides binding to MHC molecules. *Bioinformatics* **19**: 309–10.
22. Yusim, K., Korber, B.T.M., Brander, C., Haynes, B.F., Koup, R., et al. (2009) *HIV Molecular Immunology 2009*. Los Alamos National Laboratory, Theoretical Biology and Biophysics, Los Alamos, New Mexico. LA-UR 09-05941.
23. Toseland, C.P., Clayton, D.J., McSparron, H., Hemsley, S.L., Blythe, M.J., et al. (2005) AntiJen: a quantitative immunology database integrating functional, thermodynamic, kinetic, biophysical, and cellular data. *Immunome Res.* **1**: 4.
24. Blythe, M.J., Doytchinova, I.A. and Flower, D.R. (2002) JenPep: a database of quantitative functional peptide data for immunology. *Bioinformatics* **18**: 434–9.
25. Lata, S., Bhasin, M. and Raghava, G.P. (2009) MHCBN 4.0: a database of MHC/TAP binding peptides and T-cell epitopes. *BMC Res. Notes* **2**: 61.
26. Bhasin, M., Singh, H. and Raghava, G.P. (2003) MHCBN: a comprehensive database of MHC binding and non-binding peptides. *Bioinformatics* **19**: 665–6.
27. Huang, J. and Honda, W. (2006) CED: a conformational epitope database. *BMC Immunol.* **7**: 7.
28. Olah, M., Mracec, M., Ostopovici, L., Rad, R., Bora, A., et al. (2004). WOMBAT: world of molecular bioactivity. In: Oprea, T.I. (ed.) *Chemoinformatics in drug discovery*. Wiley-VCH, New York.
29. Goto, S., Okuno, Y., Hattori, M., Nishioka, T. and Kanehisa, M. (2002) LIGAND: database of chemical

Published by Woodhead Publishing Limited, 2013

compounds and reactions in biological pathways. *Nucleic Acids Res.* **30**: 402–4.

30. Irwin, J.J. and Shoichet, B.K. (2004) ZINC – a free database of commercially available compounds for virtual screening. *J. Chem. Inf. Model.* **45**: 177–82.
31. Wishart, D.S., Knox, C., Guo, A.C., Shrivastava, S., Hassanali, M., et al. (2006) DrugBank: a comprehensive resource for in silico drug discovery and exploration. *Nucleic Acids Res.* **34**: D668–72.
32. Chen, J., Swamidass, S.J., Dou, Y., Bruand, J. and Baldi, P. (2005) ChemDB: a public database of small molecules and related chemoinformatics resources. *Bioinformatics* **21**: 4133–9.

Published by Woodhead Publishing Limited, 2013

4

Database design

DOI: 10.1533/9781908818416.47

Abstract: The availability of quality data plays an important role in a successful vaccine discovery campaign. Often, this information is electronically stored in databases. The nature and complexity of a database can vary significantly, from a simple boutique database tailored to a small number of users to a large warehouse for storing tens of thousands of sequences. Database design produces a detailed blueprint of a database. It may take time, but the benefits are numerous. A well-designed database not only helps avoid redundant data, but can also provide you with access to quality, up-to-date and accurate information. It is important to understand the functions the database is expected to perform, the contents to be stored, and the concepts and features that are used to represent this information. Care should be taken to accurately model this information because it can be time-consuming to change the database structure after it is implemented. Here, we introduce you to the basic concepts of relational database design.

Key words: database design, entity-relationship model, entity-relationship diagram, normalization, normal form.

Published by Woodhead Publishing Limited, 2013

4.1 Fundamentals of database design

The relational approach to database management was first introduced by Edgar F. Codd in 1969 while working for IBM. In this model, data is organized in a series of unordered tables that can be subsequently manipulated using non-procedural queries that return tables.

4.1.1 Table

A database table is used to represent objects in the real world. In the relational model, a table consists of a series of horizontal rows and vertical columns or fields, with the cell being the point of intersection between a row and a column. Each column represents a set of data values of a particular type, while each row contains a set of related data that adheres to the same structure within the table. For example, a column in a table describing MHC peptides may contain information on the binding affinities of peptides in the database, while a row in the same table may contain, in addition to binding affinities, information on the biological assay and publication information.

4.1.2 Primary key

A primary key in a relational table is an attribute or a combination of attributes that uniquely identifies a record in the table. It can be a normal attribute that is unique in nature, such as the HLA nomenclature, or it can be a unique identifier generated by the database management system, such as a running number.

Published by Woodhead Publishing Limited, 2013

4.1.3 Foreign key

A foreign key in a relational table is a field that references a candidate key in another table. It serves as a link between data stored in two tables and can be used to join together multiple tables in a database.

4.1.4 Domain

A domain describes the set of possible values for a given attribute. For example, the data value of "IC50" is in the integer domain and not in the character domain. As such, the number "10 000" would be a possible value for the attribute "IC50" but not the words "ten thousand."

4.1.5 Relationships

Several types of relationships can be defined in a relational database.

- One-to-one relationships – a relationship that is single-valued in both directions. In a relational database, two tables share a one-to-one relationship if every row in the first table is linked to at most one row in the second table.
- One-to-many relationships – a relationship that is single-valued in one direction and multi-valued in the other. In a relational database, this occurs when each row in the first table can be linked to multiple rows in the second table but each row in the second table is linked to only one row in the first table.
- Many-to-one relationships – a relationship that is multi-valued in one direction and single-valued in the other. In a relational database, this occurs when each row in the first

Published by Woodhead Publishing Limited, 2013

table is linked to only one row in the second table but each row in the second table can be linked to multiple rows in the first table.

- Many-to-many relationships – a relationship that is multi-valued in both directions is a many-to-many relationship. Two tables in a relational database share a many-to-many relationship when every row in each table can be linked to multiple rows in the other table.

4.2 ER diagram

Entity-relationship (ER) models were first proposed by Peter Chen in 1976 as a basis to unify different views of data: the network model, the relational model, and the entity set model. They are now commonly used in software engineering to identify the stakeholders in a development process and their relationships with one another. ER diagrams are visual representations of the ER models, using conventions that describe each entity in the network and the relationships between entities. For example, the elements MHC, peptide, and pathogen may be described using the ER diagram shown in Figure 4.1. See Figure 4.2 for ER diagram symbols and notations.

There are three basic elements in an ER diagram: entity, attribute, and relationship. From these, more elements can be derived, including weak entity, multi-valued attribute, derived attribute, weak relationship, and recursive relationship.

4.2.1 Connector

A connector is a linker between an entity and an attribute, and between two attributes.

Published by Woodhead Publishing Limited, 2013

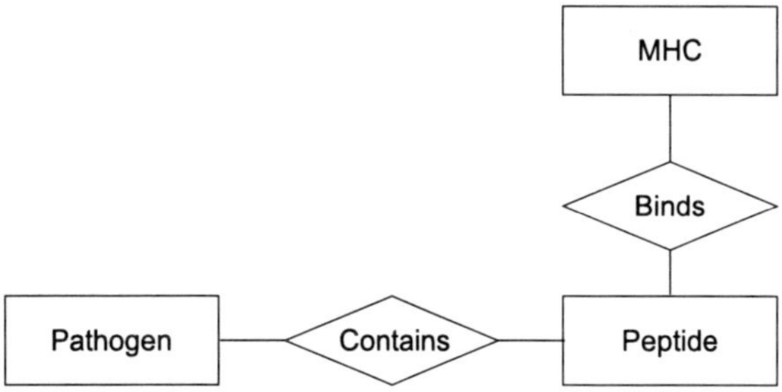

Figure 4.1 Example of a simple ER diagram depicting the relationships between MHC, peptide, and pathogen. Each entity is represented by an element within a rectangle, while the relationships between entities are represented by the items inside the diamonds

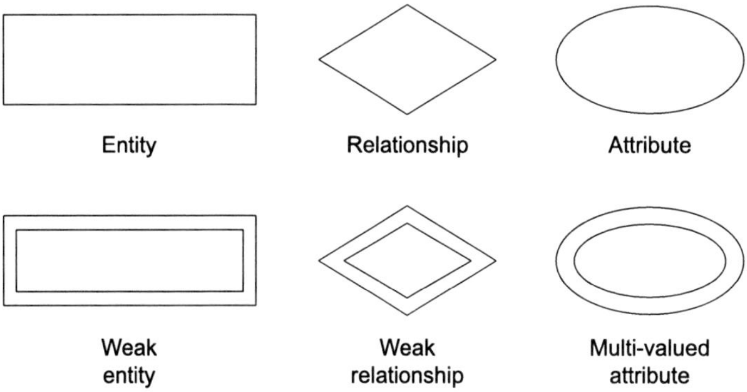

Figure 4.2 ER diagram symbols and notations

4.2.2 Entity

An entity represents an object that is present in the database. For example, it could be a molecule such as a protein, peptide, or drug, or a pathogen such as influenza A or dengue virus.

Published by Woodhead Publishing Limited, 2013

4.2.3 Weak entity

A weak entity is an entity that depends on another entity for existence and cannot be identified by its attributes alone. Such an entity uses a foreign key together with its attributes to form a primary key. A good example of this is an epitope, whose existence depends on the presence of a peptide (see Figure 4.3).

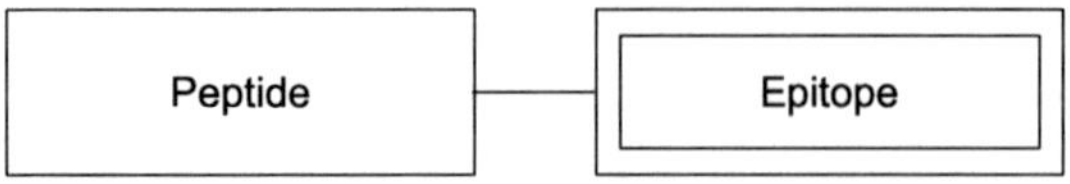

Figure 4.3 Example of a weak entity "Epitope" connected to an entity "Peptide" in an ER diagram

4.2.4 Attribute

An attribute refers to a property or characteristic of an entity, a relationship, or another attribute. This is shown in an ER diagram as an oval-shaped symbol. For example, "Physicochemical property" is an attribute of the entity "Peptide." An entity can have many attributes, and each attribute may in turn have its own attributes. For example, "Charge," "Size," "Weight," and "Polarity" are all attributes of the attribute "Physicochemical property" (see Figure 4.4).

4.2.5 Multi-valued attribute

A multi-valued attribute is an attribute that can have multiple values. This is shown as a double oval-shaped symbol in an ER diagram (see Figure 4.5). For example, the entity "Peptide" can bind to many "MHC" entities representing different class I and II alleles.

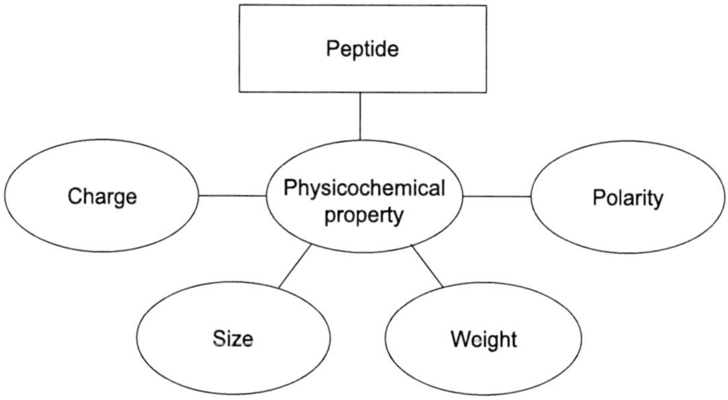

Figure 4.4 Example of attributes in an ER diagram

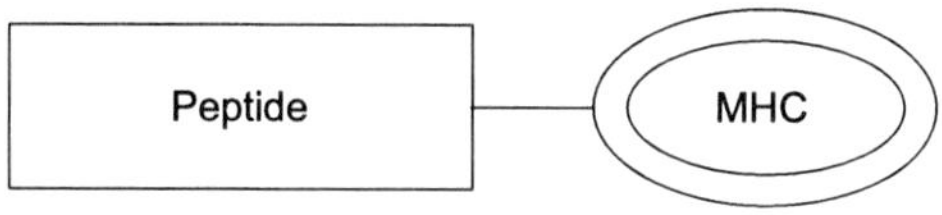

Figure 4.5 Example of a multi-valued attribute in an ER diagram

4.2.6 Relationship

A relationship in an ER diagram is used to describe the meaningful association between two entities. This is represented by a diamond-shaped symbol and labeled with a verb. For example, the entity "Pathogen" may be related to the entity "Peptide" by the relationship "Contains" (see Figure 4.6).

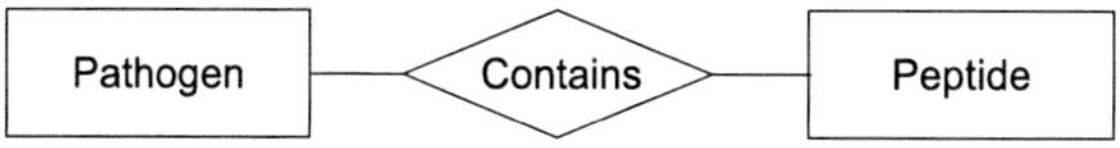

Figure 4.6 Example of a relationship between two entities in an ER diagram

Published by Woodhead Publishing Limited, 2013

4.2.7 Weak relationship

A weak relationship is a relationship that is used to connect a weak entity with others. This is represented by a double diamond-shaped symbol in an ER diagram.

4.3 Normalization and normal forms

Normalization is a logical design method that minimizes data dependency and eliminates redundant data in a relational database. A good design can help reduce disk space, ensure that data is logically stored, and improve application performance. In an un-normalized design, three problems can occur when working with the data:

- Insert anomaly – this occurs when certain data cannot be inserted into the database without the presence of other data.
- Delete anomaly – this occurs when certain data are lost unintentionally when deleting other data.
- Update anomaly – this occurs when updating the data of a column leads to database inconsistencies.

To ensure that databases are normalized, a series of guidelines have been developed by the database community. These are referred to as normal forms, numbered from one (first normal form or 1NF) through five (fifth normal form or 5NF), that decompose the data into smaller, related tables. The higher the normal form applicable to a table, the less vulnerable it is to logical inconsistencies and anomalies. These normalization guidelines are cumulative. For a database to be in 2NF, it must first fulfill all the criteria of a 1NF database.

Published by Woodhead Publishing Limited, 2013

4.3.1 First normal form (1NF)

First normal form (1NF) simplifies the attributes and sets the primary rules for an organized database. In relational terms, a table is in 1NF if it contains no duplicate columns. To convert a database to 1NF, you should:

- Remove repeating columns from the same table.
- Create individual tables for each group of related data and identify each row with a unique column or set of columns.

4.3.2 Second normal form (2NF)

Second normal form (2NF) further addresses the issue of data redundancy. For a table to be in 2NF, all of its attributes must be functionally dependent on the primary key of that table. To create a relational database that adheres to 2NF, you should:

- Ensure that the database meets all the requirements of 1NF.
- Ensure that every attribute in each table is functionally dependent on the primary key and all non-independent attributes are moved to separate tables.
- Create relationships between these new tables and their predecessors through the use of foreign keys.

4.3.3 Third normal form (3NF)

Third normal form (3NF) goes one step further than 2NF and requires all its attributes to be transitively independent of the primary key. To create a 3NF compliant database, you should:

Published by Woodhead Publishing Limited, 2013

- Ensure that the database meets all the requirements of 2NF.
- Ensure that all non-primary key attributes are independent of other non-key attributes and depend only on the primary key.

4.3.4 Boyce–Codd normal form (BCNF)

The Boyce–Codd normal form (BCNF) or 3.5NF represents a more stringent version of 3NF with one additional requirement on functional dependency. For this, you should:

- Ensure that the database meets all the requirements of 3NF.
- Ensure that every attribute is a candidate key.

4.3.5 Fourth normal form (4NF)

Fourth normal form (4NF) imposes a further requirement on database normalization, and is more concerned with multi-valued dependency than functional dependency. To implement this, you are required to:

- Ensure that the database meets all the requirements of BCNF.
- Ensure that a given relation does not contain more than one multi-valued dependency.

4.3.6 Fifth normal form (5NF)

Fifth normal form (5NF), otherwise known as Project-join normal form (PJ/NF), aims to eliminate dependencies that

Published by Woodhead Publishing Limited, 2013

are not determined by keys. To create a 5NF compliant database, you should:

- Ensure that the database meets all the requirements of 4NF.
- Ensure that every non-trivial join dependency in the database is implied by a candidate key.

4.4 Bibliography

1. Bressan, S. and Catania, B. (2000) *Introduction to database systems*. McGraw Hill Companies, Inc., New York, USA.
2. Date, C.J., Lorentzos, N. and Darwen, H. (2002) *Temporal data and the relational model*, 1st edition. Morgan Kaufmann, San Francisco, CA, USA.
3. Date, C.J. (1999) *An introduction to database systems*, 8th edition. Addison-Wesley Longman, Boston, MA, USA.
4. Elmasri, R. and Navathe, S.B. (2003) *Fundamentals of database systems*, 4th edition. Addison-Wesley, Boston, MA, USA.
5. Kent, W. (1983) A simple guide to five normal forms in relational database theory. *Commun. ACM* **26**, 120–5.
6. Ramakrishnan, R. and Gerke, J. (2002) *Database management systems*, 3rd edition. McGraw Hill Companies, Inc., New York, USA.

Published by Woodhead Publishing Limited, 2013

5

Computational T cell vaccine design

DOI: 10.1533/9781908818416.59

Abstract: T cell vaccines contain subsequences of an antigen that can induce protective T cell responses in the body. This type of vaccine is generally safer than live, attenuated vaccine, which may undergo secondary mutation in the body and revert to a virulent form. T cell vaccines can also stimulate a stronger immune response than inactivated vaccines, since they contain the specific parts of the antigen that can be recognized by T cells. However, identifying the antigens that best stimulate T cell responses is non-trivial. More than 7000 HLA alleles are deposited in the IMGT/HLA Database. Since an individual may possess up to six different HLA class I and class II alleles, the theoretical number of HLA haplotypes is more than 10^{12}. Because most binding peptides are nine amino acids long, the number of peptide candidates exceeds 10^{11}. The immune system's diversity, the complexity of its regulatory pathways, and the variability of pathogen products call for new approaches to T cell vaccine research. In this chapter, we survey MHC ligand prediction technologies.

Key words: MHC ligand prediction, T cell epitope prediction, sequence-based methods, structure-based methods, peptide-based clustering, MHC clustering.

Published by Woodhead Publishing Limited, 2013

5.1 Sequence-based methods

5.1.1 Binding motifs

Computational T cell vaccine design began in 1991 when peptide motifs were first identified in MHC class I antigens by Hans-Georg Rammensee's group in Germany. Although our knowledge of MHC–peptide interactions is still far from complete at this time, it is nevertheless sufficient for us to design rules to describe the observed binding of MHC molecules to class I and II antigens.

The engagement of MHC molecules with antigenic peptides is allele-specific, that is, each MHC molecule has its own binding preferences for the nature of peptides that can be presented in the groove. In general, these peptides are functionally related and contain amino acid residues with similar physicochemical properties at various positions of their primary sequences. Most class I and II binding peptides contain residues with side-chains that extend into polymorphic cavities (or "pockets") and bind to complementary residues of specific MHC alleles. These residues play an important role in binding interactions by "anchoring" peptides firmly at specific positions in the MHC binding cleft.

A simple approach to MHC ligand prediction would thus involve looking for key amino acid motifs in a set of MHC ligands that could serve as anchor residues, auxiliary anchors, or residues that are generally preferred by the MHC allele. To do this, one could use a measure of similarity to compute the degree of conservation of residues at each position along the primary sequence of a set of MHC ligands. The occurrence of conserved residues at each position of the peptide at a specific identity level could then be used to construct a ligand binding motif for the specific MHC allele.

Published by Woodhead Publishing Limited, 2013

Subsequent discovery showed that motifs are important, but not the sole determinants of peptide binding. Ruppert, Sidney, Celis, Kubo, Grey and Sette investigated the role of motifs in A*0201 binding (see Figure 5.1) and found that

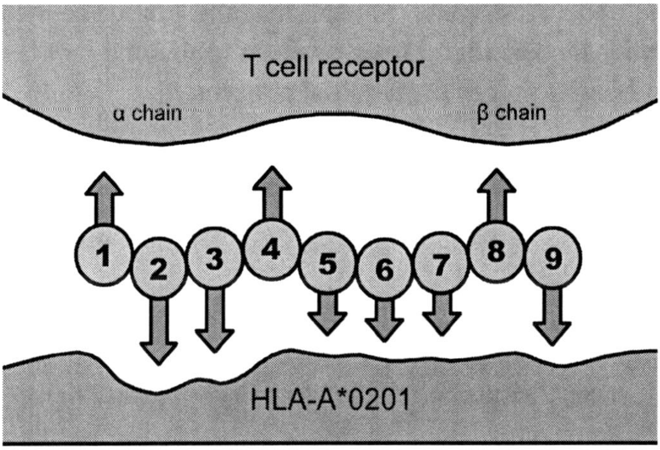

	1	2	3	4	5	6	7	8	9
anchors or *auxiliary* anchors									
		L				*V*			**V**
		M							**L**
preferred residues									
				E				K	
				K					
other residues									
	I		A	G	I	I	A	E	
	L		Y	P	K	L	Y	S	
	F		F	D	Y	T	H		
	K		P	T	N				
	M		M		G				
	Y		S		F				
	V		R		V				
					H				

Figure 5.1 Schematic diagram of HLA-A*0201 binding site showing the orientation of bound peptide residues and position-specific binding motif derived from the SYFPEITHI database

Published by Woodhead Publishing Limited, 2013

only about 30% of motif-conforming peptides were actual binders. Peptides that could achieve immunodominant status without the required binding motifs were identified, and not all motif-conforming peptides were capable of binding to the respective MHC alleles. In practice, simple motif models are both non-sensitive and non-specific, and cannot be used to identify binders that do not conform to existing motifs and non-binders that fit the required patterns.

Web resources: MHC ligand binding motifs

1. SYFPEITHI
   http://www.syfpeithi.de/
2. MHC Motif Viewer
   http://www.cbs.dtu.dk/biotools/MHCMotifViewer/Home.html
3. IEDB
   http://www.iedb.org

5.1.2 Binding matrices

Binding matrices quantify residue contributions to binding by correlating the occurrences of individual amino acid residues in a set of ligands with their positions along the primary sequence. The core of this methodology is the use of two-dimensional tables structured as rows and columns which contain $l \times 20$ coefficients, where l corresponds to the length of the set of peptides under investigation and 20 is for each of the naturally occurring amino acids (see Figure 5.2). Each cell within the table represents the individual contribution of one particular amino acid residue at a specific position within the peptide sequence to MHC binding events.

Published by Woodhead Publishing Limited, 2013

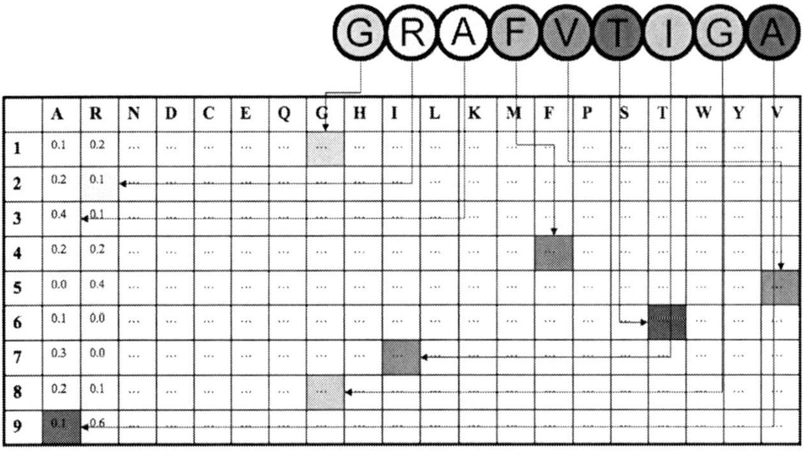

Figure 5.2 Example of a simple matrix for 9-mer peptides binding to a HLA allele. Each column represents the position of amino acid residues in the peptide and each row represents each of the 20 naturally occurring amino acids. Each cell represents the contribution of the respective amino acid at the specific position to the HLA binding event

Consensus scores are then obtained by summing, multiplying, or averaging the matrix coefficients and compared against a predetermined threshold.

In general, matrices are constructed using the position-specific frequency of amino acids along the primary sequences of known binders or quantitative MHC-binding data. The former indicates the binding likelihood of a peptide sequence to the MHC molecule, while the latter provides a means of quantifying the peptide binding affinity. The online SYFPEITHI web server and the commercial EpiMatrix software are examples of matrices based on simple counting of amino acid frequencies at different positions of known peptide binders, while BioInformatics and Molecular Analysis Section (BIMAS) was developed using peptide

Published by Woodhead Publishing Limited, 2013

binding coefficients derived from half-time dissociation rates of MHC–peptide complexes.

Attempts to detect weak binding patterns and to account for noisy and collinear data have also been reported. One example is the use of Gibbs sampler by Nielsen and colleagues to calculate weight matrices from a set of pre-aligned sequences, followed by pseudo-count correction for low counts and sequence weighting to identify potential MHC binding peptides. Another example is the use of multivariate statistics to improve the predictive performance of binding matrices. This method utilizes an additive equation to account for individual residue contributions at each position and their interactions with neighboring amino acids. Partial least squares regression is then used to produce the weight matrices. The stabilized matrix method (SMM) by Peters and Sette is a powerful predictor for HLA-A2 binding peptides. SMM consists of a matrix that describes independent amino acid contributions to binding. It is then combined with pair coefficients to quantify the impact of pairwise interactions between peptide positions.

Web resources: MHC ligand binding matrices

1. SYFPEITHI
   http://www.syfpeithi.de/
2. BIMAS
   http://www-bimas.cit.nih.gov/molbio/hla_bind/
3. SMM
   http://tools.immuneepitope.org/analyze/html/mhc_binding.html
4. MHCPred
   http://www.ddg-pharmfac.net/mhcpred/MHCPred/

Published by Woodhead Publishing Limited, 2013

5.1.3 Decision trees

Decision trees are decision support models that classify patterns using a sequence of well-defined rules. They are tree-like graphs in which each branch node represents an option between a number of alternatives, and each leaf node represents an outcome of the cumulative choices. To apply decision trees to predict MHC binding peptides, position-specific binding motifs are first converted into a series of rules. Each rule is then embedded within the nodes of a tree. The resulting tree structure indicates amino acid properties that are strongly correlated with the physicochemical properties of binding peptides. Peptide sequences can then be threaded through a series of nodes, and the results of all node-to-node transitions are used to infer their binding specificities. An example of a decision tree network is shown in Figure 5.3.

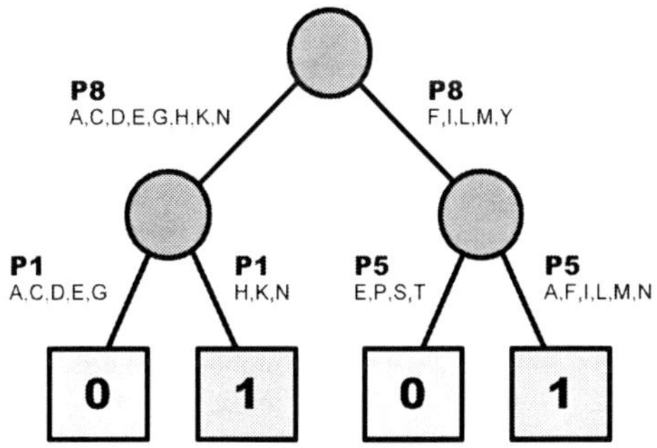

Figure 5.3 Subset of a simple decision tree network. Binding motifs are converted into rules and embedded within the nodes of a tree. Predicted outcome is represented by 0 (non-binding) or 1 (binding) at each node. Ellipses and rectangles represent internal and terminal nodes respectively

Published by Woodhead Publishing Limited, 2013

5.1.4 Artificial neural networks

An artificial neural network (ANN) is a connectionist model that is inspired by the way biological neural networks process information. It consists of an interconnected group of artificial neurons working in parallel to solve specific problems. Here, a single artificial neuron is a single node in a directed graph, with one or more input connections and a single output connection. To form a network, several nodes are connected, with the output of some providing the input of others. Some nodes receive inputs from the external world to feed the internal nodes; some nodes are "hidden" and do not interact directly with outside; and others deliver the output from the network to the external world. See example in Figure 5.4.

To apply ANNs for MHC ligand prediction, the first step is to extract features from the sequence data set and convert them into a series of numerical descriptors. Example features

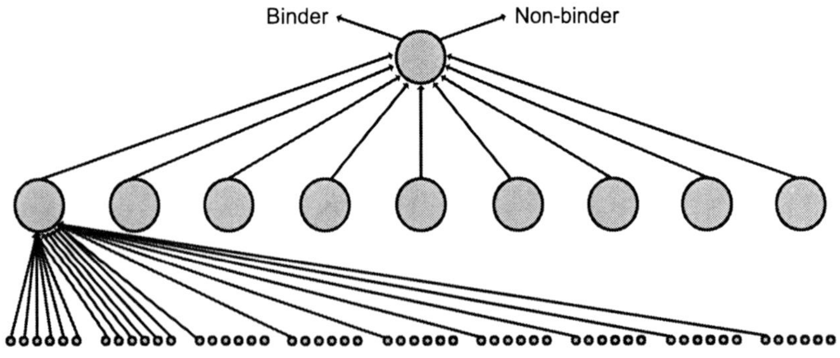

Figure 5.4 Example of a three-layer ANN commonly used for predicting HLA class I 9-mer peptides. The first layer is the input nodes corresponding to the length of the input peptide; the second (i.e. hidden) layer corresponds to the ideal length of binding peptides; and the third (i.e. output) layer is a single node that predicts binding or non-binding

Published by Woodhead Publishing Limited, 2013

could be the physicochemical properties of amino acids, such as composition, charge, hydrophobicity, polarity, and volume. The descriptors are used as input to train an ANN classifier to recognize the patterns of binding. An ANN takes as input a fixed number of source nodes. As such, existing ANN models are mostly trained to predict binding peptides that are of the same length as those in the training data set. This restricts the ability to predict epitopes with lengths that differ from those used in the trained network. In the context of MHC binding predictions, studies have shown that the performance of ANNs gradually outperforms motifs, matrices, and hidden Markov models (HMMs) with increasing peptide data. They are commonly used in MHC binding predictions, for high-throughput screening of class I and II antigens at both allele-specific and superfamily level.

Web resources: ANN predictors

1. NetMHCpan
   http://www.cbs.dtu.dk/services/NetMHCpan/
2. NetMHCIIpan
   http://www.cbs.dtu.dk/services/NetMHCIIpan/
3. MULTIPRED2
   http://cvc.dfci.harvard.edu/multipred2/index.php
4. IEDB-AR
   http://tools.immuneepitope.org/analyze/html/mhc_binding.html

5.1.5 Support vector machines

A support vector machine (SVM) is a statistical learning method based on the structural risk minimization principle.

Published by Woodhead Publishing Limited, 2013

It uses the concept of decision planes that utilize decision boundaries to optimally separate data into different categories. Similar to the ANN method, every peptide sequence is first represented by specific feature vector assembled from encoded representations of residue properties such as amino acid composition, hydrophobicity, polarity, charge, bulkiness, and solvent accessibility. The parameters of SVM are then calibrated, first by mapping the input vectors into a high-dimensional space, followed by maximizing the margin between the binders and non-binders with an optimal separating hyperplane. Similar to decision tree, ANN, and HMM, SVM has the ability to handle both linear and non-linear data. This method outperforms ANN and decision tree in the absence of a large training data set and has been very widely used in MHC binding predictions.

Web resources: SVM predictors

1. MHC2Pred
   http://imtech.res.in/raghava/mhc2pred/
2. SVMHC
   http://abi.inf.uni-tuebingen.de/Services/SVMHC

5.1.6 Hidden Markov models

A hidden Markov model (HMM) is a probabilistic graphical model that is commonly used in statistical pattern recognition and classification. It is a powerful tool for detecting weak signals, and has been successfully applied in temporal pattern recognition such as speech, handwriting, word sense disambiguation, and computational biology.

Published by Woodhead Publishing Limited, 2013

A HMM consists of two components. Each HMM contains a series of discrete-state, time-homologous, first-order Markov chains (MC) with suitable transition probabilities between states and an initial distribution. A MC is a discrete-time process for which the next state is conditionally independent of the past given the current state. Each state has a discrete or continuous probability distribution over possible emissions or outputs. These outputs are generated when a particular state is visited or during transition from one state to another. State-to-state transitions are guided by a set of transition and emission probabilities. The transition probability is the probability of moving from one state to another via a connected edge, and the emission probability is the probability of emitting a particular symbol at a state. The sequences of states through which the model passes are hidden and cannot be observed, hence the name hidden Markov model. The probability of any sequence, given the model, is computed by multiplying the emission and transition probabilities along the path.

HMM topologies that have been used for MHC ligand prediction include profile HMM and fully connected HMM. A profile HMM (Figure 5.5(a)) is a linear left-right model where the underlying directed graph is acyclic, with the exception of loops, hence supporting a partial order of the states. The profile HMM architecture contains three classes of states: the match state, the insert state, and the delete state; and two sets of parameters: transition probabilities and emission probabilities. The match and insert states always emit a symbol, whereas the delete states are silent states without emission probabilities. A fully connected HMM (Figure 5.5(b)) consists of states that are pairwise connected such that the underlying digraph is complete. There are no distinguished starting and terminating states, and the transition matrix does not contain any zero entries,

Published by Woodhead Publishing Limited, 2013

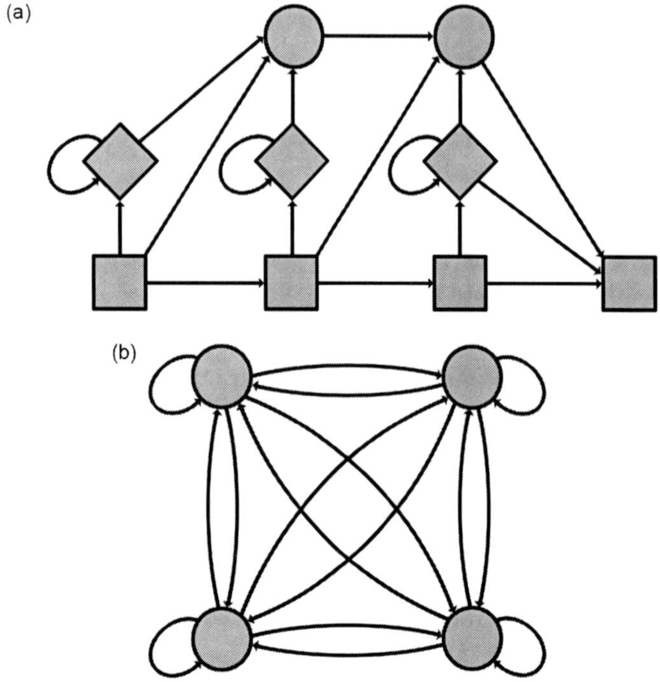

Figure 5.5 **Example of HMM topologies used for predicting HLA class I binding peptides: a) a profile HMM, b) a fully connected HMM**

with the exception of diagonal entries, which correspond to loops or self-transitions. Because there is no constraint on the structure of a fully connected HMM, this model permits the representation of more than one sequence pattern hidden in the training data.

5.2 Structure-based methods

5.2.1 Protein threading

Protein threading or side-chain conformational search is a method commonly used for fold recognition. The basic idea

Published by Woodhead Publishing Limited, 2013

of this method is to compare a target MHC–peptide sequence against a library of known structures and see how well each potential structure would fit the sequence. The highest-ranking structure is then assumed to best fit the fold of the target complex.

Steps in protein threading are:

1. Align the amino acid sequence of the target MHC–peptide complex with that of a known structure.
2. Substitute the side-chains of the source peptide (P_1, P_2, . . . P_n) that is bound to a MHC molecule of interest with the target peptide sequence (S_1, S_2, . . . S_n) by replacing P_i with S_i.
3. Replace the side-chains of residues in the source MHC molecule if it differs from the target MHC sequence.
4. Refine the stereochemical quality of the model by limited energy minimization.
5. Score the model using energy potentials, knowledge-based rules, similarity indices, and/or other methods to discriminate binders from non-binders.

Margalit and colleagues applied this technique for peptides binding to A*0201, Aw68, B*2705, B*3501, B*5301, B*0801, H-2K^b, H-2D^b, and H-2M3 using the statistical pairwise potential table of Miyazawa and Jernigan. It successfully identified peptides binding to MHC molecules with hydrophobic binding pockets but not to MHC molecules with hydrophilic, charged pockets. To solve this problem, other scoring methods were introduced, including the use of other knowledge-based potentials that described hydrophilic interactions more appropriately, and similarity indices derived from 3D quantitative structure–affinity relationship (QSAR) studies.

Published by Woodhead Publishing Limited, 2013

5.2.2 Homology modeling

Homology modeling or comparative modeling employs the use of available homologous protein structure(s) to predict the unknown structure of a related amino acid sequence. The aim is to model the bound conformation of a MHC–peptide sequence given the 3D structure of other bound peptides to homologous MHC molecules. It is the direct opposite of protein threading techniques, in that it computes how well each sequence fits a structure rather than vice versa.

Steps in homology modeling are as follows:

1. Select the template structure from a database of known structures (e.g. PDB) using sequence similarity searches. The Basic Local Alignment Search Tool (BLAST) is a commonly used algorithm for finding suitable templates.
2. Align the amino acid sequence of the target MHC–peptide complex with that of the selected template.
3. Construct a set of models by satisfaction of spatial restraints using the MODELLER software. The model returning with the least restraints is selected for further analysis.
4. Refine the stereochemical quality of the model by limited energy minimization.
5. Assess the model to ensure that there are no atomic clashes using software such as WHAT IF and Ramachandran plot.

Several groups have used this method to characterize TCR/peptide/MHC and peptide/MHC interactions and MHC associations with disease. For example, Hammer and coworkers constructed a series of synthetic peptide/HLA-DRB1*0402 models from HA peptide/HLA-DRB1*0101 crystallographic structure to study its correlation with

Published by Woodhead Publishing Limited, 2013

rheumatoid arthritis. Michielin and Karplus applied the technique to identify critical residues of the A6 TCR that interacts with peptide/HLA-A2 complex. Almagro and colleagues constructed a model of 5C.C7/MCC 93-103/I-Ek to study the structural role for TCR a1, a2, b1, and b2 in MHC interaction. A framework was subsequently proposed to create testable hypotheses about TCR recognition.

5.2.3 Molecular docking

Molecular docking or computer-simulated ligand binding is a powerful technique for investigating intermolecular interactions. In general, the goals of docking are two-fold:

1. To assess the relative goodness-of-fit of the peptide. This is to identify the most probable position and orientation of a peptide within the MHC binding groove. MHC class I and II molecules are well characterized with six (A to F) and nine (1–9) pockets in the peptide-binding grooves, respectively. In this context, the basis of docking is to identify the most probable complementation in size, shape, and intermolecular forces of a given MHC–peptide pair. A complication for MHC class II molecules is the open nature of the binding groove. A single peptide may have multiple binding registers (i.e. core residues) that interact with a given receptor. In such cases, the binding modes of all possible core residues should be analyzed.
2. To assess the affinity of the peptide to the target MHC molecule. A scoring function is commonly used to rank peptides. Three classes of scoring functions are commonly used in a docking campaign – force field-based methods, empirical scoring functions and knowledge-based potentials. Force field-based methods use classical molecular dynamics to calculate the binding free energies

Published by Woodhead Publishing Limited, 2013

of MHC–peptide complexes. These are estimated by the sum of van der Waals and electrostatic interactions. Empirical scoring functions estimate binding free energies using weighted structural parameters obtained by fitting the scoring functions to experimental binding constants of a set of complexes. Knowledge-based scoring functions are based on the number of observed intermolecular interactions between the receptor–ligand pair. The simplicity of this method allows rapid screening of large data sets.

5.3 Broad-based T cell vaccine design

The design of T cell vaccine with wide population coverage is a strategy that has been gaining popularity over the past decade. The goal is to identify MHC alleles that are present in most individuals from all major ethnic groups, and to ensure that they can bind to at least one peptide in the vaccine cocktail. In this respect, two related concepts may be the ones that provide the solution – promiscuous peptides that bind more than one HLA allele; and MHC superfamilies that represent sets of molecules with largely overlapping binding specificities.

5.3.1 Peptide-based clustering

One way to identify promiscuous T-cell epitopes is to define clusters of peptide specificities according to their MHC alleles. A clustering procedure for MHC class I peptides by Lund and colleagues works as follows:

1. Given a set of peptide sequences, construct a 9-mer alignment of sequences for each MHC allele and estimate

Published by Woodhead Publishing Limited, 2013

the best scoring pattern in terms of highest relative entropy.

2. Construct a weight matrix that represents the specificity of the MHC molecule using the equation $\log(p_{ap}/q_a)$, where p_{ap} is the estimated frequency of amino acid a at position p in the alignment and q_a the background frequency of amino acid a in the SwissProt database.
3. Calculate the distance between each pair of matrices using the equation $d_{ij} = \Sigma_a(1 - (p^i_a \bullet p^j_a) / (|p^i_a|\,|p^j_a|))$, where p^i_a and p^j_a are the vectors of 20-amino-acid frequencies at position p in matrix i and j respectively. Normalize the distance matrix by dividing all distances with $d_{ij}^{\max}$.
4. Cluster the distance matrices using a neighbor-joining algorithm such as those implemented in PHYLIP, MATLAB, or R.
5. Perform bootstrap analysis to estimate the significance of the clustering outcome.
6. Now we have a set of binding motifs that can be visualized using sequence logo programs.

5.3.2 MHC clustering

MHC supertypes or MHC alleles with similar binding specificities share common structural features within the MHC binding groove. The concept of MHC supertypes was first introduced by Sette's group at the La Jolla Institute for Allergy and Immunology in 1996, based on peptide motifs and simple structural analyses. A commonly used method to identify such alleles is to look for structural similarities of their binding pockets. Flower and colleagues used this method to study the binding pockets of HLA-A, -B, -C, -DR, -DQ, and -DP alleles. The procedure includes:

Published by Woodhead Publishing Limited, 2013

1. Extraction of binding site residues from 3D structures of MHC–peptide complexes.
2. Comparative molecular similarity index analysis (CoMSIA) of the 3D structures. The generated properties include: steric bulk, electrostatic potential, hydrophobicity, and hydrogen-bond donor and acceptor abilities.
3. Generation of molecular interaction field (MIF) descriptors from the HLA binding site using particular probes, using software such the Molecular Discovery GRID program.
4. Principal component analysis (PCA) of the MIF descriptors to uncover differences in the binding sites with respect to their probe interaction pattern.

5.4 Bibliography

1. Falk, K., Rötzschke, O., Stevanović, S., Jung, G. and Rammensee, H.G. (1991) Allele-specific motifs revealed by sequencing of self-peptides eluted from MHC molecules. *Nature* **351**: 290–6.
2. Sidney, J., Oseroff, C., del Guercio, M.F., Southwood, S., Krieger, J.I., et al. (1994) Definition of a DQ3.1-specific binding motif. *J. Immunol.* **152**: 4516–25.
3. Parker, K.C., Bednarek, M.A. and Coligan, J.E. (1994) Scheme for ranking potential HLA-A2 binding peptides based on independent binding of individual peptide side-chains. *J. Immunol.* **152**: 163–75.
4. Hammer, J., Bono, E., Gallazzi, F., Belunis, C. and Sinigaglia, F. (1994) Precise prediction of major histocompatibility complex class II-peptide interaction based on peptide side chain scanning. *J. Exp. Med.* **180**: 2353–8.

Published by Woodhead Publishing Limited, 2013

5. Rammensee, H.G., Friede, T. and Stevanovic, S. (1995) MHC ligands and peptide motifs: first listing. *Immunogenetics* **41**: 178–228.
6. Rapin, N., Hoof, I., Lund, O. and Nielsen, M. (2008) MHC motif viewer. *Immunogenetics* **60**: 759–65.
7. Meister, G.E., Roberts, C.G.P., Berzofsky, J.A. and De Groot, A.S. (1995) Two novel T cell epitope prediction algorithms based on MHC-binding motifs; comparison of predicted and published epitopes from Mycobacterium tuberculosis and HIV protein sequences. *Vaccine* **13**: 581–91.
8. D'Amaro, J., Houbiers, J.G.A., Drijfhout, J.W., Brandt, R.M., Schipper, R., et al. (1995) A computer program for predicting possible cytotoxic T lymphocyte epitopes based on HLA class I peptide-binding motifs. *Hum. Immunol.* **43**: 13–18.
9. Peters, B. and Sette, A. (2005) Generating quantitative models describing the sequence specificity of biological processes with the stabilized matrix method. *BMC Bioinformatics* **6**: 132.
10. Rajapakse, M., Schmidt, B. and Brusic, V. (2006) *Multi-objective evolutionary algorithm for discovering peptide binding motifs*, 4th European Workshop on Evolutionary Computation and Machine Learning in Bioinformatics (EvoBIO 2006), Budapest, Hungary, Springer, LNCS 3907, 149–58.
11. Chen, W., Khilko, S., Fecondo, J., Margulies, D.H. and McCluskey, J. (1994) Determinant selection of major histocompatibility complex class I-restricted antigenic peptides is explained by class I-peptide affinity and is strongly influenced by nondominant anchor residues. *J. Exp. Med.* **180**: 1471–83.
12. Jameson, S.C. and Bevan, M.J. (1992) Dissection of major histocompatibility complex (MHC) and T cell

Published by Woodhead Publishing Limited, 2013

receptor contact residues in a Kb-restricted ovalbumin peptide and an assessment of the predictive power of MHC-binding motifs. *Eur. J. Immunol.* **22**: 2663–7.

13. Ruppert, J., Sidney, J., Celis, E., Kubo, R.T., Grey, H.M., et al. (1993) Prominent role of secondary anchor residues in peptide binding to HLA-A2.1 molecules. *Cell* **74**: 929–37.
14. Martin, W., Sbai, H. and De Groot, A.S. (2003) Bioinformatics tools for identifying class I-restricted epitopes. *Methods* **29**: 289–98.
15. Yu, K., Petrovsky, N., Schonbach, C., Koh, J.Y.L. and Brusic, V. (2002) Methods for prediction of peptide binding to MHC molecules: a comparative study. *Mol. Med.* **8**: 137–48.
16. Davenport, M.P., Ho Shon, I.A.P. and Hill, A.V.S. (1995) An empirical method for the prediction of T-cell epitopes. *Immunogenetics* **42**: 392–7.
17. Gulukota, K., Sidney, J., Sette, A. and DeLisi, C. (1997) Two complementary methods for predicting peptides binding major histocompatibility complex molecules. *J. Mol. Biol.* **267**: 1258–67.
18. Schafer, J.R., Jesdale, B.M., George, J.A., Kouttab, N.M. and De Groot, A.S. (1998) Prediction of well-conserved HIV-1 ligands using a matrix-based algorithm, EpiMatrix. *Vaccine* **16**: 1880–84.
19. Reche, P.A., Glutting, J.P. and Reinherz, E.L. (2002) Prediction of MHC class I binding peptides using profile motifs. *Hum. Immunol.* **63**: 701–9.
20. Peters, B., Tong, W., Sidney, J., Sette, A. and Weng, Z. (2003) Examining the independent binding assumption for binding of peptide epitopes to MHC-I molecules. *Bioinformatics* **19**: 1765–72.
21. Nielsen, M., Lundegaard, C., Worning, P., Hvid, C.S., Lamberth, K., et al. (2004) Improved prediction of

Published by Woodhead Publishing Limited, 2013

MHC class I and class II epitopes using a novel Gibbs sampling approach. *Bioinformatics* **20**: 1388–97.
22. Rajapakse, M., Wyse, L., Schmidt, B. and Brusic, V. (2005) Deriving matrix of peptide-MHC interactions in diabetic mouse by genetic algorithm. *Lecture Notes in Computer Science* **3578**: 440–7.
23. Guan, P., Doytchinova, I.A., Zygouri, C. and Flower, D.R. (2003) MHCPred: bringing a quantitative dimension to the online prediction of MHC binding. *Appl. Bioinformatics* **2**: 63–6.
24. Guan, P., Doytchinova, I.A. and Flower, D.R. (2003) HLA-A3 supermotif defined by quantitative structure–activity relationship analysis. *Protein Eng.* **16**: 11–18.
25. Doytchinova, I.A., Blythe, M.J. and Flower, D.R. (2002) Additive method for the prediction of protein-peptide binding affinity. Application to the MHC Class 1 molecule HLA-A*0201. *J. Proteome Res.* **1**: 263–72.
26. Duda, R.O., Hart, P.E. and Stork, D.G. (2001) *Pattern classification*. New York: Wiley-Interscience.
27. Savoie, C.J., Kamikawaji, N., Sasazuki, T. and Kuhara, S. (1999) Use of BONSAI decision trees for the identification of potential MHC class I peptide epitope motifs. *Pac. Symp. Biocomput.* 182–9.
28. Segal, M.R., Cummings, M.P. and Hubbard, A.E. (2001) Relating amino acid sequence to phenotype: analysis of peptide-binding data. *Biometrics* **57**: 632–42.
29. Zurada, J.M. (1999) *Introduction to Artificial Neural Systems*. St Paul, MN, USA: PWS Publishing Co.
30. Brusic, V., Rudy, G. and Harrison, L.C. (1994) Prediction of MHC binding peptides using artificial neural networks. In: Stonier, R.J. and Yu, X.S. (eds) *Complex Systems: Mechanism of Adaptation*. Amsterdam: IOS Press, 253–60.

Published by Woodhead Publishing Limited, 2013

31. Brusic, V., Rudy, G., Honeyman, M., Hammer, J. and Harrison, L. (1998) Prediction of MHC class II-binding peptides using an evolutionary algorithm and artificial neural network. *Bioinformatics* **14**: 121–30.
32. Nielsen, M., Lundegaard, C., Justesen, S., Lund, O. and Buus, S. (2010) NetMHCIIpan-2.0 – Improved pan-specific HLA-DR predictions using a novel concurrent alignment and weight optimization training procedure. *Immunome Res.* **6**: 9.
33. Zhang, G.L., Deluca, D.S., Keskin, D.B., Chitkushev, L., Zlateva, T., et al. (2011) MULTIPRED2: a computational system for large-scale identification of peptides predicted to bind to HLA supertypes and alleles. *J. Immunol. Methods* **374**: 53–61.
34. Adams, H.P. and Koziol, J.A. (1995) Prediction of binding to MHC class I molecules. *J. Immunol. Methods* **185**: 181–90.
35. Milik, M., Sauer, D., Brunmark, A.P., Yuan, L., Vltiello, A., et al. (1998) Application of an artificial neural network to predict specific class I MHC binding peptide sequences. *Nat. Biotechnol.* **16**: 753–6.
36. Buus, S. (1999) Description and prediction of peptide-MHC binding: the human MHC project. *Curr. Opin. Immunol.* **11**: 209–13.
37. Nielsen, M., Lundegaard, C., Worning, P., Lauemøller, S. L., Lamberth, K., et al. (2003) Reliable prediction of T-cell epitopes using neural networks with novel sequence representations. *Protein Sci.* **12**: 1007–17.
38. Han, L.Y., Cai, C.Z., Ji, Z.L., Cao, Z.W. and Chen, Y.Z. (2004) Predicting functional family of novel enzymes irrespective of sequence similarity: a statistical learning approach. *Nucleic Acids Res.* **32**: 6437–44.
39. Zhao, Y., Pinilla, C., Valmori, D., Martin, R. and Simon, R. (2003) Application of support vector

machines for T-cell epitopes prediction. *Bioinformatics* **19**: 1978–84.

40. Dönnes, P. and Elofsson, A. (2002) Prediction of MHC class I binding peptides, using SVMHC. *BMC Bioinformatics* **3**: 25.
41. Rabiner, L.R. (1989) A tutorial on hidden Markov models and selected applications in speech recognition. *Proc. IEEE* **77**: 257–86.
42. Mamitsuka, H. (1989) Predicting peptides that bind to MHC molecules using supervised learning of hidden Markov models. *Proteins* **33**: 460–74.
43. Durbin, R., Eddy, S., Krogh, A. and Mitchison, G. (1998) *Biological Sequence Analysis: Probabilistic Models of Proteins and Nucleic Acids*. Cambridge: Cambridge University Press, 51–68.
44. Akutsu, T. and Sim, K.L. (1999) Protein threading based on multiple protein structure alignment. *Genome Inform*. **10**: 23–9.
45. Sezerman, U., Vajda, S. and DeLisi, C. (1996) Free energy mapping of class I MHC molecules and structural determination of bound peptides. *Protein Sci.* **5**: 1272–81.
46. Altuvia, Y., Schueler, O. and Margalit, H. (1995) Ranking potential binding peptides to MHC molecules by a computational threading approach. *J. Mol. Biol.* **249**: 244–50.
47. Miyazawa, S. and Jernigan, R.L. (1985) Estimation of effective inter-residue contact energies from protein crystal structures: quasi-chemical approximation. *Macromolecules* **18**: 534–52.
48. Miyazawa, S. and Jernigan, R.L. (1996) Residue-residue potentials with a favorable contact pair term and an unfavorable high packing density term, for simulation and threading. *J. Mol. Biol.* **256**: 623–44.

Published by Woodhead Publishing Limited, 2013

49. Altuvia, Y., Sette, A., Sidney, J., Southwood, S. and Margalit, H. (1997) A structure-based algorithm to predict potential binding peptides to MHC molecules with hydrophobic binding pockets. *Hum. Immunol.* **58**: 1–11.
50. Schueler-Furman, O., Elber, R. and Margalit, H. (1998) Knowledge-based structure prediction of MHC class I bound peptides: a study of 23 complexes. *Fold. Des.* **3**: 549–64.
51. Kangueane, P., Sakharkar, M.K., Lim, K.S., Hao, H., Lin, K., et al. (2000) Knowledge-based grouping of modeled HLA peptide complexes. *Hum. Immunol.* **61**: 460–6.
52. Schueler-Furman, O., Altuvia, Y., Sette, A. and Margalit, H. (2000) Structure-based prediction of binding peptides to MHC class I molecules: application to a broad range of MHC alleles. *Protein Sci.* **9**: 1838–46.
53. Betancourt, M.R. and Thirumalai, D. (1999) Pair potentials for protein folding: choice of reference states and sensitivity of predicted native states to variations in the interaction schemes. *Protein Sci.* **8**: 361–9.
54. Jojic, N., Reyes-Gomez, M., Heckerman, D., Kadie, C. and Schueler-Furman, O. (2006) Learning MHC I-peptide binding. *Bioinformatics* **22**: e227–35.
55. Bui, H.H., Schiewe, A.J., von Grafenstein, H. and Haworth, I.S. (2006) Structural prediction of peptides binding to MHC class I molecules. *Proteins* **63**: 43–52.
56. Doytchinova, I.A. and Flower, D.R. (2001) Toward the quantitative prediction of T-cell epitopes: coMFA and coMSIA studies of peptides with affinity for the class I MHC molecule HLA-A*0201. *J. Med. Chem.* **44**: 3572–81.
57. Swindells, M.B. and Thornton, J.M. (1991) Structure prediction and modelling. *Curr. Opin. Biotechnol.* **2**: 512–19.

Published by Woodhead Publishing Limited, 2013

58. Sali, A. and Blundell, T.L. (1993) Comparative protein modeling by satisfaction of spatial restraints. *J. Mol. Biol.* **234**: 774–815.
59. Rognan, D., Laumoeller, S.L., Holm, A., Buus, S. and Tschinke, V. (1999) Predicting binding affinities of protein ligands from three-dimensional models: application to peptide binding to class I major histocompatibility proteins. *J. Med. Chem.* **42**: 4650–8.
60. Logean, A., Sette, A. and Rognan, D. (2001) Customized versus universal scoring functions: application to class I MHC-peptide binding free energy predictions. *Bioorg. Med. Chem. Lett.* **11**: 675–9.
61. Michielin, O., Luescher, I. and Karplus, M. (2000) Modeling of the TCR-MHC-peptide complex. *J. Mol. Biol.* **300**: 1205–35.
62. Michielin, O. and Karplus, M. (2002) Binding free energy differences in a TCR-peptide-MHC complex induced by a peptide mutation: a stimulation analysis. *J. Mol. Biol.* **324**: 547–69.
63. Almagro, J.C., Vargas-Madrazo, E., Lara-Ochoa, F. and Horjales, E. (1995) Molecular modeling of a T-cell receptor bound to a major histocompatibility complex molecule: Implications for T-cell recognition. *Protein Sci.* **4**: 1708–11.
64. Rosenfeld, R., Zheng, Q., Vajda, S. and DeLisi, C. (1993) Computing the structure of bound peptides: Application to antigen recognition by class I major histocompatibility complex receptors. *J. Mol. Biol.* **234**: 515–21.
65. Rosenfeld, R., Zheng, Q., Vajda, S. and DeLisi, C. (1995) Flexible docking of peptides to class I major-histocompatibility-complex receptors. *Genet. Anal.* **12**: 1–21.

Published by Woodhead Publishing Limited, 2013

66. Lim, J.S., Kim, S., Lee, H.G., Lee, K.Y., Kwon, T.J., et al. (1996) Selection of peptides that bind to the HLA-A2.1 molecule by molecular modelling. *Mol. Immunol.* 33: 221–30.
67. Antes, I., Siu, S.W. and Lengauer, T. (2006) DynaPred: a structure and sequence based method for the prediction of MHC class I binding peptide sequences and conformations. *Bioinformatics* **22**: e16–24.
68. Bordner, A.J. and Abagyan, R. (2006) Ab initio prediction of peptide-MHC binding geometry for diverse class I MHC allotypes. *Proteins* **63**: 512–26.
69. Tong, J.C., Tan, T.W. and Ranganathan, S. (2004) Modeling the structure of bound peptide ligands to major histocompatibility complex. *Protein Sci.* **13**: 2523–32.
70. Tong, J.C., Bramson, J., Kanduc, D., Chow, S., Sinha, A.A., et al. (2006) Modeling the bound conformation of pemphigus vulgaris-associated peptides to MHC class II DR and DQ alleles. *Immunome Res.* **2**:1.
71. Tong, J.C., Zhang, G.L., Tan, T.W., August, J.T., Brusic, V., et al. (2006) Prediction of HLA-DQ3.2b ligands: evidence of multiple registers in class II binding peptides. *Bioinformatics* **22**: 1232–8.
72. Ramachandran, G.N., Ramakrishnan, C. and Sasisekharan, V. (1963) Stereochemistry of polypeptide chain configurations. *J. Mol. Biol.* 7: 95–9.
73. Vriend, G. (1990) WHAT IF: a molecular modeling and drug design program. *J. Mol. Graph.* **8**: 52–6.
74. Hammer, J., Gallazzi, F., Bono, E., Karr, R.W., Guenot, J., et al. (1995) Peptide binding specificity of HLA-DR4 molecules: correlation with rheumatoid arthritis association. *J. Exp. Med.* 181: 1847–55.
75. Michielin, O. and Karplus, M. (2002) Binding free energy differences in a TCR-peptide-MHC complex

induced by a peptide mutation: a stimulation analysis. *J. Mol. Biol.* **324**: 547–69.
76. Almagro, J.C., Vargas-Madrazo, E., Lara-Ochoa, F. and Horjales, E. (1995) Molecular modeling of a T-cell receptor bound to a major histocompatibility complex molecule: implications for T-cell recognition. *Protein Sci.* **4**: 1708–11.
77. Breda, A., Basso, L.A., Santos, D.S. and de Azevedo Jr, W.F. (2008) Virtual screening of drugs: scoring functions, docking and drug design. *Curr. Comput. Aided Drug Des.* **4**: 265–72.
78. Sturniolo, T., Bono, E., Ding, J., Raddrizzani, L., Tuereci, O., et al. (1999) Generation of tissue-specific and promiscuous HLA ligand databases using DNA microarrays and virtual HLA class II matrices. *Nat. Biotechnol.* **17**: 555–61.
79. Brusic, V., Petrovsky, N., Zhang, G. and Bajic, V.B. (2002) Prediction of promiscuous peptides that bind HLA class I molecules. *Immunol. Cell. Biol.* **80**: 280–5.
80. Lund, O., Nielsen, M., Kesmir, C., Petersen, A.G., Lundegaard, C., et al. (2004) Definition of supertypes for HLA molecules using clustering of specificity matrices. *Immunogenetics* **12**: 797–810.
81. Saitou, N. and Nei, M. (1987) The neighbor-joining method: a new method for reconstructing phylogenetic trees. *Mol. Biol. Evol.* **4**: 406–25.
82. Doytchinova, I.A., Guan, P. and Flower, D.R. (2004) Identifying human MHC supertypes using bioinformatic methods. *J. Immunol.* **172**: 4314–23.
83. Doytchinova, I.A. and Flower, D.R. (2005) In silico identification of supertypes for class II MHCs. *J. Immunol.* **174**: 7085–95.

Published by Woodhead Publishing Limited, 2013

84. Kangueane, P., Sakharkar, M.K., Rajaseger, G., Bolisetty, S., Sivasekari, B., et al. (2005) A framework to sub-type HLA supertypes. *Front. Biosci.* **10**: 879–86.
85. Zhao, B., Png, A.E.H., Ren, E.C., Kolatkar, P.R., Mathura, V.S., et al. (2003) Compression of functional space in HLA-A sequence diversity. *Hum. Immunol.* **64**: 718–28.
86. Sidney, J., Grey, H.M., Kubo, R.T. and Sette, A. (1996) Practical, biochemical and evolutionary implications of the discovery of HLA class I supermotifs. *Immunol. Today* **17**: 261–6.

Published by Woodhead Publishing Limited, 2013

6

Computational B cell vaccine design

DOI: 10.1533/9781908818416.87

Abstract: The ability to predict B cell epitopes accurately remains an unsolved problem in computational immunology. One of the biggest challenges is the lack of standards in defining B cell epitopes, which has a direct impact on the selection and development of appropriate tools for analysis. Most B cell epitopes vary from five to more than 20 amino acids in length. About 90% of B cell epitopes are non-contiguous in nature. Some of the amino acids are in contact with the immunoglobulin, while others may be located far from the protein surface. Some amino acid residues are essential for binding the immunoglobulin, while others may not be functionally important. Due to these inherent complexities, development of highly accurate B cell epitope prediction systems is difficult. Here, we survey the specialized tools and methods for the modeling and prediction of B cell epitopes. The goal is to provide you with better understanding of the strengths and limitations of current techniques.

Key words: B cell epitope prediction, sequence-based methods, structure-based methods, computational immunology, propensity assessment, machine learning, feature mapping, substructure search.

Published by Woodhead Publishing Limited, 2013

6.1 Sequence-based methods

6.1.1 Propensity scales

Propensity scales represent one of the earliest methods used to map B cell epitopes. The principle of these methods is simple: certain amino acid physicochemical properties are frequently found on antigenic determinants. By assigning a propensity value to each amino acid in a protein based on these observed properties, the scores can be used to predict whether a given residue is part of an epitope sequence. For example, charged, hydrophilic and solvent-exposed amino acid residues are common features of B cell epitopes. It might be possible that some of these epitopes are associated with stretches of amino acid sequence with high concentration of charged and polar residues, and are lacking in large hydrophobic residues. Hopp and Woods investigated this first in 1981, and introduced the use of the Levitt hydrophilicity scale to locate protein antigenic determinants. Over the years, other propensity scales have been proposed by various groups, including:

- Jameson and Wolf's antigenic index, which includes parameters for surface accessibility, regional backbone flexibility, and predicted secondary structure.
- Emini's solvent accessibility score, which is based on Janin and Wodak's surface accessibility scale on surface exposure probabilities for amino acids computed using the X-ray crystallographic structures of 28 proteins.
- Karplus and Schulz's flexibility scale, which describes segmental flexibility using the temperature factors (i.e. B-values) of C_α atoms from 31 protein structures.
- Kolaskar's antigenic scale, using the antigenic propensity of residues derived from 156 antigenic determinants in 34 proteins.

Published by Woodhead Publishing Limited, 2013

- Parker's hydrophobicity scale, which was derived from high-performance liquid chromatography (HPLC) peptide retention data on a reversed-phase column.
- Pellequer's turn scale, which is based on the occurrence of amino acids at each of the four positions of a turn using a set of 87 protein structures.

Despite their popularity in B cell epitope mapping, the effectiveness of propensity scales has so far been controversial. In 2005, Blythe and Flower assessed the predictive performance of 484 amino acid propensity scales from the Amino Acid Index Database (Aaindex; *http://www.genome.jp/aaindex/*) for B cell epitope prediction and found that the best set of scales and parameters performed only slightly better than random.

Web resources: Propensity assessment algorithms

1. ProtScale
   http://web.expasy.org/protscale/
2. IEDB Analysis Resource
   http://tools.immuneepitope.org/tools/bcell/iedb_input
3. Bcepred
   http://www.imtech.res.in/raghava/bcepred/

6.1.2 Machine learning techniques

Just like their T cell counterparts, machine learning techniques are heavily applied in predicting both linear and conformational B cell epitopes. The descriptors used to train these algorithms could be derived from amino acid sequences,

Published by Woodhead Publishing Limited, 2013

from a combination of propensity scales such as hydrophilicity, flexibility, polarity, and exposed surface, amino acid composition, or from structural properties extracted from 3D models.

Computationally, it is hard to predict B cell epitopes, more so for conformational ones, due to their highly variable length and the low level of homology between epitope sequences. So far this approach has not achieved a sufficient level of accuracy for the desired practical application. The area under the receiver operating characteristic curve (A_{ROC}) is a commonly used measure to assess the performance of predictive methods. A ROC curve is a graphical plot of true positive rate (i.e. sensitivity) against false positive rate (i.e. 1 – specificity) for a binary classifier system across different discrimination thresholds. An A_{ROC} of 0.5 reflects random forecasts, while an A_{ROC} of 1.0 represents perfect tests. If the estimated A_{ROC} is less than 0.5, it indicates that the test's performance is worse than chance. In summary, the A_{ROC} provides an overall summary of the predictive accuracy. For most of the existing B cell epitope predictors, their A_{ROC} hover around 0.6.

Web resources: Machine learning algorithms

4. ABCpred – linear epitopes
   Artificial neural network
   http://www.imtech.res.in/raghava/abcpred/
5. BCPREDS – linear epitopes
   Support vector machine
   http://ailab.cs.iastate.edu/bcpreds/
6. BepiPred – linear epitopes
   Hidden Markov model and propensity scales
   http://www.cbs.dtu.dk/services/BepiPred/

Published by Woodhead Publishing Limited, 2013

7. CBTOPE – non-linear epitopes
   Support vector machine
   http://www.imtech.res.in/raghava/cbtope/index.php
8. Epitopia – linear and non-linear epitopes
   Naïve Bayes classifier
   http://epitopia.tau.ac.il/

6.2 Structure-based methods

Structure-based methods are more powerful and robust for mapping B cell epitopes. Such methods can perform high-complexity computations and are better at describing spatial information. Over the past decade, these methods are gaining dominance, due to:

- the rapidly increasing number of 3D structures of antibody–antigen complexes in the PDB and in IMGT/3Dstructure-DB;
- the ability to predict both linear and non-linear epitopes.

Because the success of this method depends on the quality of the 3D model used, it is important to know this quality before the start of a screening campaign.

6.2.1 Feature mapping

Feature mapping is a common method for predicting non-linear B cell epitopes. If the residues of a conformational epitope are not contiguous in primary sequence but are brought into spatial proximity by protein folding, the surface properties and composition of known protein structures can serve as the basis for epitope prediction. A typical feature

Published by Woodhead Publishing Limited, 2013

mapping method would take a 3D model of a protein, determine its local or global surface characteristics, such as solvent accessibility, relative accessible surface area, B-factor value (i.e. mobility of protein backbones), side-chain orientation, charges, polarity, hydrophobicity or hydrophilicity, and use the information as the basis for epitope discrimination. A candidate epitope sequence would be a region along the primary sequence that has a high concentration of the particular surface characteristics. Where multiple surface characteristics are used, a predictive score may be assigned to each residue to indicate the likelihood that it is an epitope residue. A simple scoring system for ranking candidate sequences can be developed using a linear combination of the descriptors used.

Web resources: Feature mapping techniques

1. DiscoTope – non-linear epitopes
   http://www.cbs.dtu.dk/services/DiscoTope/
2. BEpro (formerly known as PEPITO) – non-linear epitopes
   http://pepito.proteomics.ics.uci.edu/info.html
3. CEP – linear and non-linear epitopes
   http://115.111.37.205/cgi-bin/cep.pl
4. SEPPA – non-linear epitopes
   http://lifecenter.sgst.cn/seppa/index.php
5. ElliPro – non-linear epitopes
   http://tools.immuneepitope.org/tools/ElliPro/

6.2.2 Substructure search

A related concept is the use of substructure similarity search techniques to identify surface contours on proteins

Published by Woodhead Publishing Limited, 2013

that are conserved among B cell epitope sequences. This method can combine physicochemical properties of amino acid residues with geometrical conformations to perform the search. A clique is a subset of a graph where every two vertices in the subset are connected by an edge. A maximum clique is a clique with the largest size in a graph. (See Figure 6.1 for an example of a maximum clique problem.) In current practice, the query and target protein structures are represented as graphs, and the goal is to find the maximum common subgraphs of the input graphs. This can be done by transforming the input graphs into an edge-product graph, and finding the maximum clique(s) or fully connected subgraph(s) in the edge-product graph. Alternatively, a weight can be assigned to each node to represent amino acid similarity (e.g. solvent accessible surface area) between query residues and graph vertices. A scoring function can then be used to rank the candidate substructures, for example, using the amino acid similarity weights or the root mean square deviation (RMSD) criterion.

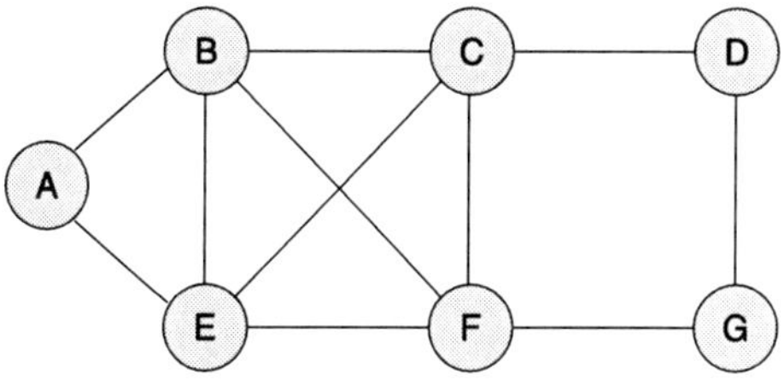

Figure 6.1 Example of a maximum clique problem. The set {A, B, E} forms a clique. The set {B, C, E, F} forms the maximum clique. The set {C, D, F, G} is not a clique as vertices C and G, and vertices D and F, are not joined by an edge

Published by Woodhead Publishing Limited, 2013

> ***Web resources:*** Substructure search
>
> 1. Pepitope
>   *http://pepitope.tau.ac.il/*

6.3 Bibliography

1. Hopp, T.P. and Woods, K.R. (1981) Prediction of protein antigenic determinants from amino acid sequences. *Proc. Natl. Acad. Sci. USA* **78**: 3824–8.
2. Pellequer, J.L., Westhof, E. and Van Regenmortel, M.H. (1991) Predicting location of continuous epitopes in proteins from their primary structure. *Meth. Enzymol.* **203**: 176–201.
3. Pellequer, J., Westhof, E. and Van Regenmortel, M. (1993) Correlation between the location of antigenic sites and the prediction of turns in proteins. *Immunol. Lett.* **36**: 83–99.
4. Emini, E., Hughes, J., Perlow, D. and Boger, J. (1985) Induction of hepatitis A virus-neutralizing antibody by a virus-specific synthetic peptide. *J. Virol.* **55**: 836–9.
5. Jameson, B.A. and Wolf, H. (1988) The antigenic index: a novel algorithm for predicting antigenic determinants. *Comput. Appl. Biosci.* **4**: 181–6.
6. El-Manzalway, Y. and Honavar, V. (2010) Recent advances in B-cell epitope prediction methods. *Immunome Res.* **6**: S2.
7. Levitt, M. (1976) A simplified representation of protein conformations for rapid simulation of protein folding. *J. Mol. Biol.* **104**: 59–107.

Published by Woodhead Publishing Limited, 2013

8. Saha, S. and Raghava, G.P. (2006) Prediction of continuous B-cell epitopes in an antigen using recurrent neural network. *Proteins* **65**: 40–8.
9. Haste Andersen, P., Nielsen, M. and Lund, O. (2006) Prediction of residues in discontinuous B-cell epitopes using protein 3D structures. *Protein Sci.* **15**: 2558–67.
10. Parker, J. and Guo, H.R.D. (1986) New hydrophilicity scale derived from high-performance liquid chromatography peptide retention data: correlation of predicted surface residues with antigenicity and x-ray-derived accessible sites. *Biochemistry* **25**: 5425–32.
11. Karplus, P. and Schulz, G. (1985) Prediction of chain flexibility in proteins: a tool for the selection of peptide antigen. *Naturwiss.* **72**: 212–13.
12. Blythe, M. and Flower, D. (2005) Benchmarking B cell epitope prediction: underperformance of existing methods. *Protein Sci.* **14**: 246–8.
13. Kawashima, S. and Kanehisa, M. (2000) AAindex: Amino acid index database. *Nucleic Acids Res.* **28**: 374.
14. Janin, J. and Wodak, S. (1978) Conformation of amino acid side-chains in proteins. *J. Mol. Biol.* **125**: 357–86.
15. Rost, B. and Sander, C. (1994) Conservation and prediction of solvent accessibility in protein families. *Proteins* **20**: 216–26.
16. Zhang, W., Xiong, Y., Zhao, M., Zou, H., Ye, X., et al. (2011) Prediction of conformational B-cell epitopes from 3D structures by random forests with a distance-based feature. *BMC Bioinformatics* **12**: 341.
17. Liu, R. and Hu, J. (2011) Prediction of discontinuous B-cell epitopes using logistic regression and structural information. *J. Proteomics Bioinform.* **4**: 11–15.
18. Sun, J., Wu, D., Xu, T., Wang, X., Xu, X., et al. (2009) SEPPA: a computational server for spatial epitope

Published by Woodhead Publishing Limited, 2013

prediction of protein antigens. *Nucleic Acids Res.* **37**: W612–16.

19. Sweredoski, M.J. and Baldi, P. (2008) PEPITO: improved discontinuous B-cell epitope prediction using multiple distance thresholds and half sphere exposure. *Bioinformatics* **24**: 1459–60.
20. Saha, S. and Raghava, G.P.S. (2004) BcePred: Prediction of continuous B-cell epitopes in antigenic sequences using physico-chemical properties. In: Nicosia, G., Cutello, V., Bentley, P.J. and Timis, J. (eds) ICARIS 2004, LNCS 3239: 197–204.
21. Kulkarni-Kale, U., Bhosle, S. and Kolaskar, A.S. (2005) CEP: a conformational epitope prediction server. *Nucleic Acids Res.* **33**: W168–71.
22. Ansari, H.R. and Raghava, G.P.S. (2010) Identification of conformational B-cell epitopes in an antigen from its primary sequence. *Immunome Res.* **6**: 6.
23. Rubinstein, N.D., Mayrose, I., Martz, E. and Pupko, T. (2009) Epitopia: a web-server for predicting B-cell epitopes. *BMC Bioinformatics* **10**: 287.
24. Ponomarenko, J., Bui, H.-H., Li, W., Fusseder, N., Bourne, P.E., et al. (2008) ElliPro: a new structure-based tool for the prediction of antibody epitopes. *BMC Bioinformatics* **9**: 514.
25. Kolaskar, A.S. and Tongaonkar, P.C. (1990) A semi-empirical method for prediction of antigenic determinants on protein antigens. *FEBS* **276**: 172–4.
26. Odorico, M. and Pellequer, J.L. (2003) BEPITOPE: predicting the location of continuous epitope and patterns in proteins. *J. Mol. Recognit.* **16**: 20–2.
27. Aung, Z. and Tong, J.C. (2008) BSAlign: a rapid graph-based algorithm for detecting ligand-binding sites in protein structures. *Genome Inform.* **21**: 65–76.

Published by Woodhead Publishing Limited, 2013

28. Mayrose, I., Shlomi, T., Rubinstein, N.D., Gershoni, J.M., Ruppin, E., et al. (2007) A graph-based algorithm for epitope mapping using combinatorial phage-display libraries. *Nucleic Acid Res.* 35: 69–78.
29. Bublil, E.M., Freund, N.T., Mayrose, I., Penn, O., Roitburd-Berman, A., et al. (2007) Stepwise prediction of conformational discontinuous B-cell epitopes using the Mapitope algorithm. *Proteins* 68: 294–304.

Published by Woodhead Publishing Limited, 2013

7

Infectious disease informatics

DOI: 10.1533/9781908818416.99

Abstract: Throughout history, infectious diseases have posed a serious burden to mankind. More recently, there has been an alarming increase in drug-resistant microbes. Furthermore, new pathogens are emerging due to microbial evolution and adaptation. The spread of these diseases is a result of pathogen mutations and changes in human behavior patterns. Then, there are diseases that are lurking in the background, waiting for the right conditions before they strike again. In the war against these diseases, we have come to understand the behaviors of microbes in a heterogeneous world and the mechanisms governing disease transmission. These works have profoundly shaped modern knowledge of emerging and re-emerging infections. More recently, computational techniques have led the way into this new era by allowing rapid high-throughput analysis of pathogens which was previously not possible using traditional laboratory techniques. This chapter introduces methods in mathematical modeling, computational biology, and bioinformatics that have been used to study infectious diseases.

Key words: infectious disease modeling, infectious disease informatics, sequence analysis, information entropy, molecular evolution.

Published by Woodhead Publishing Limited, 2013

7.1 Infectious diseases in history

Epidemics, pandemics, and outbreaks of infectious diseases are regular features of life on earth. In 430 BC, Thucydides described the very first pandemic in recorded history – the Athenian plague that reportedly killed up to one-half of the citizens of Athens. In AD 541–2, an outbreak occurred in the Byzantine Empire, causing 10 000 deaths every day. The outbreak, named the Justinian plague after the reigning emperor Justinian I, resulted in over 100 million deaths and wiped out nearly half the inhabitants of the city. In 1348–50, the plague returned to Europe under the name of the Black Death, killing up to 60% of the continent's population. In March 1918, an influenza outbreak was first reported in a US military camp in Kansas. The outbreak, later known as the "Spanish flu," subsequently spread and infected up to a billion people, or half the world's population at the time, causing some 50 million deaths within six months. All over the world, changes in socio-economic, demographic and environmental factors brought about by urbanization and industrialization have led to the resurgence of old and new infectious diseases.

Over the past 40 years, there has been an alarming increase in drug-resistant microbes in diseases such as malaria and tuberculosis. Furthermore, the world is also witnessing the emergence of more new pathogens due to microbial evolution and adaptation. These include the Marburg virus in 1967, Lassa fever virus in 1969, rotavirus in 1973, Ebola virus in 1976, human immunodeficiency virus (HIV) in 1981, hepatitis C virus (HCV) in 1989, hantavirus in 1993, and the severe acute respiratory syndrome coronavirus (SARS-CoV) in 2002. The spread of these diseases is a result of pathogen mutations and changes in human behavior patterns, including lifestyles, environmental degradation, travel, and drug use.

Published by Woodhead Publishing Limited, 2013

Then, there are diseases that are lurking in the background, waiting for the right conditions before they strike again. In 1999, West Nile virus re-emerged in New York and spread across the United States to Long Island, Connecticut, Maryland, Florida, California, Arizona, and Colorado, with over 4100 reported cases and 280 associated deaths within a span of five years. Previously known to be a mild disease, the re-emergence of epidemic Chikungunya virus (CHIKV) in Africa, Indian Ocean, South-East Asia, Pacific, North America, and Europe in the past decade has caused severe morbidity with some cases of fatality. In April 2009, a new strain of human influenza A (H1N1) virus containing genes from human, swine and avian influenza A viruses emerged in Mexico. Over the course of one year, the virus had spread to more than 212 countries and overseas territories or communities, causing more than 15 921 deaths. More recently, in January 2012, a human case of avian influenza A (H5N1) virus infection was reported in China. If history is our guide, we can assume that the threat of these diseases will continue to grow and pose a serious problem to the security of countries worldwide.

7.2 Microbial sequence analysis

7.2.1 Sequence alignment

Similarity between related sequences can give clues to the structure, function, or homology to the common ancestor. Computational methods that can compare sequence features are, therefore, particularly useful. Sequence alignment is the determination of residue–residue correspondences between two or more character strings, usually preserving the relative order. This method allows us to measure similarity and infer

Published by Woodhead Publishing Limited, 2013

evolutionary relationships between two or more sequences. Pairwise sequence alignment is useful for analyzing the degree of similarity between two biological sequences. Where more than two sequences are involved, multiple sequence alignment can be used to identify regions of similarity that may help explain functional and/or phenotypic variability. The 2009 H1N1 flu was not the first human pandemic caused by influenza A viruses. It is related to the 1889 Russian flu that killed ~1 million people, the 1918 Spanish flu that infected ~25% of the global population and killed at least 50 million people worldwide, the 1957 Asian flu that resulted in ~2 million deaths and the 1968 Hong Kong flu that caused ~1 million deaths. In cases where the ancestry is unclear, sequence alignment methods can be used to infer their phylogenetic relationships. This includes:

- identifying globally optimal alignment solutions for studying highly conserved sequences;
- identifying maximally homologous subsequences among sets of long sequences for detecting distantly related proteins.

In information theory and computer science, four types of metrics are commonly used to measure the edit distance between two strings of characters. They include:

- The Hamming distance, which is the number of positions with mismatched characters between two strings of the same length.
- The Levenshtein distance, which is the minimum number of operations that is needed to transform one string into the other, which may be of different length. An operation can be a deletion, insertion, or substitution of a single character in the strings.

Published by Woodhead Publishing Limited, 2013

- The Damerau-Levenshtein distance, which is the minimum number of operations that is needed to transform one string into the other, which may be of different length. An operation can be a deletion, insertion, or substitution of a single character, or a transposition of two adjacent characters in the strings.
- The Jaro-Winkler distance, which is a measure of similarity between two strings using the Jaro distance metric. This method first identifies the common characters between two strings of characters. Two characters are common if there is an exact match and if the difference in positions between the two strings is less than half the length of the shorter string. Once all the common characters are determined, the number of transpositions of common characters are determined and used to compute the Jaro similarity. Strings that are more similar will have a higher Jaro distance.

In biological systems, certain amino acid changes are more likely to occur than others. For example, a hydrophobic residue is more likely to be replaced by another hydrophobic residue than a hydrophilic residue. To account for such transformations, a weight can be assigned to the different edit operations. This can take the form of a matrix that shows the substitution frequencies of observed pairs of amino acid residues. Two popular substitution matrices are:

- The Percent Accepted Mutation (PAM) matrices by Dayhoff, which measure sequence similarity in closely related species. Two sequences 1 PAM apart have an average of one accepted point mutation event per 100 amino acids. They need not be 99% identical, as two point accepted mutations can occur at the same position. To analyze sequences that are more divergent, we can use the PAM1 matrix as a base for calculating other matrices.

Published by Woodhead Publishing Limited, 2013

This is based on the assumption that repeated mutations would follow the same pattern as those in the PAM1 matrix.

- The BLOck SUbstitution Matrix (BLOSUM) matrices by Henikoff and Henikoff, which measure sequence similarity in divergent sequences. The matrices are constructed from the BLOCKS database of aligned conserved regions in divergent protein families. These regions are assumed to be of functional importance.

Once the substitution matrix is selected, the optimal alignment can be found using dynamic programming algorithms.

7.2.2 Information entropy

A related concept is the use of theoretical statistics, such as information entropy, to quantify the rate of information transfer in biological sequences. The Shannon entropy is a measure of uncertainty that is associated with a random variable. It is commonly used to assess the variability of microbial proteomes and epitope sequences. For a given alignment, the information content (i.e. entropy) of an amino acid position $H(x)$ is defined by:

$$H(x) = -\Sigma\ P(x) \log P(x)$$

where x is one of 20 amino acid residue types. $P(x)$, the probability of occurrence of x, is estimated by $f(x)$, the frequency of the appearance of residue type within the alignment column:

$$P(x) \approx f(x) = N(x)/L$$

where $N(x)$ is the number of appearances of amino acid residue x, and L is the length of the column. This method has

Published by Woodhead Publishing Limited, 2013

been used to analyze the genetic diversity and antigenic relationships of Chikungunya virus (CHIKV) proteomes from its introduction in 1952 to 2009. Antigenic switches refer to changes in gene expression at a specific site which may abrogate binding to HLA molecules or antagonize/interfere with T cell response, leading to cellular immune evasion. The study suggested that CHIKV is undergoing mild positive selection, with significant amounts of "antigenic switches" clustered over the entire genome.

An effective way to identify amino acid residues that are involved in virus adaptation is to find interdependencies between mutations in multiple proteins. A simple way to do this is to calculate mutual information (MI) between variable pairs. MI is an information theoretical statistic that measures the strength of association between a pair of variables. The mutual information between two variables A and B is defined by:

$$MI(A, B) = H(A) + H(B) - H(A, B)$$

where $H(A)$ and $H(B)$ are entropies of A and B, while $H(A, B)$ is their joint entropy over a set of all possible unique pairs of values (A, B). This method can also be used to identify characteristic sites in pathogen proteins with conserved mutations. For example, Miotto and colleagues applied this method in 2010 to identify adaptive signatures of influenza A proteomes from 92 343 sequences.

7.3 Detecting natural selection in molecular evolution

The evolutionary inertia of a pathogen can be qualitatively examined by studying the nucleotide usage patterns at single amino acid sites. The neutral theory of molecular evolution

Published by Woodhead Publishing Limited, 2013

by Kimura in 1968 states that most evolutionary changes at the molecular level are caused by random genetic drift of selectively neutral nucleotide substitutions. Due to the degeneracy of the genetic code, some point mutations are silent with no amino acid replacements. Silent or synonymous substitutions are primarily transparent to natural selection, whereas replacement or non-synonymous substitutions may be a result of strong selective pressure. A simple method to calculate the extent of adaptive evolution at highly variable genetic loci is to compare the fixation rates between non-synonymous (d_N) and synonymous (d_S) substitutions.

The d_N/d_S ratio (ω), otherwise known as the "acceptance rate," provides a sensitive measure of selection pressure at the amino acid level. $\omega=1$ indicates neutral expectation, $\omega<1$ suggests negative (purifying) selection, while $\omega>1$ suggests positive (diversifying) selection. A group of genes that often show the $\omega>1$ relationship are antigenic genes in human immunodeficiency virus-1, plasmodia, and other parasites. The hemagglutinin gene from influenza A virus is probably one of the fastest evolving genes in terms of the rate of nucleotide substitution, which was estimated at 5.7×10^{-3} per site per year. This high genetic variation confers a fitness advantage to the pathogen in its attempt to evade host defenses.

The simple counting method of Nei and Gojobori is commonly used for estimating d_N and d_S. However, the reliability of this technique is low when the rate of transitional nucleotide change is higher than that of transversional change. The model-based maximum likelihood (ML) methods such as those proposed by Muse and Gaut and Goldman and Yang represent a viable and widely used alternative for this purpose. The original ML model of Goldman and Yang assumes a single ω for all lineages and sites, and has been extended to account for variation by

Published by Woodhead Publishing Limited, 2013

allowing ω to vary either across lineages, among substitution sites, or both among sites and among lineages. Lineage-specific models assume that ω do not vary among sites, and can detect positive selection for a lineage only if the averaged d_N over all sites is greater than the average d_S. Site-specific models, on the other hand, allow ω to vary among sites but not among lineages. As such, these models can detect positive selection at individual sites only if the averaged d_N over all lineages is greater than the average d_S. By allowing ω to vary both among sites and among lineages, the method can be applied to detect positive selection that occurred at a few time points and affects a few sites.

7.4 Bibliography

1. Kemena, C. and Notredame, C. (2009) Upcoming challenges for multiple sequence alignment methods in the high-throughput era. *Bioinformatics* **25**: 2455–65.
2. Bhattacharya, T., Daniels, M., Heckerman, D., Foley, B., Frahm, N., et al. (2007) Founder effects in the assessment of HIV polymorphisms and HLA allele associations. *Science* **315**: 1583–6.
3. Shannon, C.E. (1950) Prediction and entropy of printed English. *Bell System Technical Journal* 30, 50–64.
4. Tong, J.C., Simarmata, D., Lin, R.T.P., Renia, L. and Ng, L.F.P. (2010) HLA class I restriction as a possible driving force for Chikungunya evolution. *PLoS ONE* 5: e9291.
5. Miotto, O., Heiny, A.T., Albrecht, R., Garcia-Sastre, A., Tan, T.W., et al. (2010) Complete-proteome mapping of human influenza A adaptive mutations: implications for human transmissibility of zoonotic strains. *PLoS ONE* 5: e9025.

Published by Woodhead Publishing Limited, 2013

6. Sheng, C., Hsu, W., Lee, M.L., Tong, J.C. and Ng, S.K. (2010) Mining mutation chains in biological sequences. *Proc. Int. Conf. on Data Engineering ICDE*: 473–84.
7. Grenfell, B.T., Pybus, O.G., Gog, J.R., Wood, J.L.N., Daly, J.M., et al. (2004) Unifying the epidemiological and evolutionary dynamics of pathogens. *Science* **303**: 327–32.
8. Bennett, S.N., Holmes, E.C., Chirivella, M., Rodriguez, D.M., Beltran, M., et al. (2003) Selection-driven evolution of emergent dengue virus. *Mol. Biol. Evol.* **20**: 1650–8.
9. Suzuki, Y. and Gojobori, T. (1999) A method for detecting positive selection at single amino acid sites. *Mol. Biol. Evol.* **16**: 1315–28.
10. Suzuki, Y., Gojobori, T. and Nei, M. (2001) ADAPTSITE: detecting natural selection at single amino acid sites. *Bioinformatics* **17**: 660–1.
11. Kimura, M. (1968) Evolutionary rate at the molecular level. *Nature* **217**: 624–6.
12. Nei, M. (2005) Selectionism and neutralism in molecular evolution. *Mol. Biol. Evol.* **22**: 2318–42.
13. Miyata, T. and Yasunaga, T. (1980) Molecular evolution of mRNA: a method for estimating evolutionary rates of synonymous and amino acid substitutions from homologous nucleotide sequences and its applications. *J. Mol. Evol.* **16**: 23–36.
14. Air, G.M. (1981) Sequence relationships among the hemagglutinin genes of 12 subtypes of influenza A virus. *Proc. Natl. Acad. Sci. USA* **78**: 7639–43.
15. Nei, M. and Gojobori, T. (1986) Simple methods for estimating the numbers of synonymous and nonsynonymous nucleotide substitutions. *Mol. Biol. Evol.* **3**: 418–26.

Published by Woodhead Publishing Limited, 2013

16. Muse, S.V. and Gaut, B.S. (1994) A likelihood approach for comparing synonymous and nonsynonymous nucleotide substitution rates, with application to the chloroplast genome. *Mol. Biol. Evol.* **11**: 715–24.
17. Goldman, N. and Yang, Z. (1994) A codon-based model of nucleotide substitution for protein-coding DNA sequences. *Mol. Biol. Evol.* **11**: 725–36.
18. Kosakovsky Pond, S.L., Poon, A.F.Y., Brown, A.J.L. and Frost, S.D.W. (2008) A maximum likelihood method for detecting directional evolution in protein sequences and its application to influenza A virus. *Mol. Biol. Evol.* **25**: 1809–4.
19. Yang, Z. and Nielsen, R. (2002) Codon-substitution models for detecting molecular adaptation at individual sites along specific lineages. *Mol. Biol. Evol.* **19**: 908–17.

Published by Woodhead Publishing Limited, 2013

8

Vaccine safety and quality assessments

DOI: 10.1533/9781908818416.111

Abstract: A pharmaceutical compound must be absorbed, distributed into the tissues, metabolized by specialized enzymes and finally excreted from the body (absorption, distribution, metabolism and excretion – ADME). Genetic variability in drug metabolizing enzymes may cause toxicity in some individuals (Tox). It is therefore necessary to carry out preclinical evaluation before testing a compound in humans. Similarly to other pharmaceutical products, vaccines must be carefully assessed for their safety and effectiveness before phased trials with humans are performed. Factors such as compound size, aqueous solubility, ionizability and lipophilicity can give information on "drug-likeness," and potential allergenicity has been estimated by sequence homology of the compound with known allergens. Here, we review computational methods of ADME/Tox assessment and allergenicity prediction that can facilitate the conformance of safety and quality in vaccine research and development.

Key words: ADME/Tox assessment, drug-likeness, lead-likeness, allergenicity prediction, computational methods.

8.1 Assessment of ADME/Tox deficiencies

The disposition of a pharmaceutical compound within our body may be described by its absorption, distribution, metabolism and excretion (ADME) properties. In order to exert a pharmacological effect in tissues, a compound has to penetrate several physiological barriers, including the gastrointestinal barrier, the blood–brain barrier and the microcirculatory barrier, to reach the blood circulation. It is subsequently transported to its site of action for distribution into tissues and organs, degraded by specialized enzymes, and finally removed from the body via excretion. In addition, genetic variation in drug metabolizing enzymes implies that some compounds may undergo metabolic activation and cause adverse reactions or toxicity (Tox) in humans. Accordingly, preclinical ADME/Tox studies can help investigate the usefulness and safety of a compound.

The membrane permeability of a compound is determined by a combination of factors that include compound size, aqueous solubility, ionizability (pKa) and lipophilicity (logP). In 1997, Palm and colleagues reported that the polar surface area (PSA) of a compound has an inverse correlation with the lipid penetration ability. Compounds that are completely absorbed by humans tend to have PSA values of ≤60Å^2, while compounds with PSA >140Å^2 are less than 10% absorbed. A PSA of 120–140 Å^2 is consequently proposed as an upper limit for the design of oral compounds. Lipinski carefully studied the physico-chemical properties of 2245 drugs from the World Drug Index (WDI) and found that compounds with the following criteria are more likely to have poor absorption and permeation:

- the molecular weight (MW) is smaller than 500 Da.

Published by Woodhead Publishing Limited, 2013

- the n-octanol/water partition coefficient value (logP) is less than five.
- the number of hydrogen bond donors (HBD) is less than five.
- the number of hydrogen bond acceptors (HBA) is less than ten.

As all the above numbers are multiples of five, a "rule of five" was subsequently proposed as a metric for evaluating drug-likeness. Lipinski's rule states that an orally active drug should have no more than one violation of the above criteria. Several variants of these rules have been proposed by other researchers, including those proposed by Ghose, Viswanadhan and Wendoloski. After reviewing seven different subsets of drug molecules from the Comprehensive Medicinal Chemistry (CMC) database, the team suggested that the qualifying range of a "drug-like" compound is:

- the molecular weight is between 160 and 480 g/mol.
- the ClogP value is between −0.4 and 5.6.
- the molar refractivity is between 40 and 130.
- the total number of atoms is between 20 and 70.

A more stringent "rule of five" was also proposed by Wenlock and colleagues in 2003 after analysis of 594 compounds from the Physicians' Desk Reference 1999. The team found that most lipophilic compounds are being discontinued from development, and that orally administered drugs satisfy the following criteria:

- the molecular weight is less than 473 g/mol.
- the ClogP value is less than 5.
- the number of hydrogen bond donors is less than 4.
- the number of hydrogen bond acceptors is less than 7.

Published by Woodhead Publishing Limited, 2013

A "rule of three" for lead-likeness was also proposed by Congreve and coworkers after analysis of a range of targets derived by NMR and X-ray crystallography. In general, these fragments satisfy the following properties:

- the molecular weight is less than 300 g/mol.
- the number of hydrogen bond donors is less than or equal to 3.
- the ClogP value is less than or equal to 3.

Despite their popularity for preclinical studies, one should note that these rules can only serve as the minimal criteria for evaluating drug-likeness. It has been estimated that 68.7% of compounds in the Available Chemical Directory (ACD) Screening Database (2.4 million compounds) and 55% of compounds in ACD (240 000 compounds) do not violate the "rule of five."

8.2 Assessment of allergenicity

Allergy is an immune system response caused by adverse immunologic reaction to normally harmless substances known as allergens. The acute symptoms of allergy are usually due to the release of inflammatory mediators when an allergen cross-links IgE antibodies on mast cells or basophils. This may be followed by a late-phase reaction characterized by the influx of T cells, eosinophils and monocytes. Atopic individuals may have one or more manifestations of the disease, including asthma, conjunctivitis, dermatitis (eczema), rhinitis (hay fever), and the severe anaphylaxis.

Computational methods are now commonly used to help assess potential allergenicity in protein sequences. Early

Published by Woodhead Publishing Limited, 2013

methods relied on the use of sequence homology with known allergens. In 1996, the International Food Biotechnology Council (IFBC) and the Allergy and Immunology Institute of the International Life Sciences Institute (ILIS) developed a decision-tree approach to assess the allergenic potential of genetically engineered crop plants. This approach was highly popular with the agricultural biotechnology industry. Eventually, the method was modified by the World Health Organization (WHO) and Food and Agriculture Organization (FAO) in a joint expert consultation on foods derived from biotechnology. In the consultation report, guidelines were established for evaluating the allergenicity of genetically modified foods. In addition to biological tests on the protein of interest, a protein is considered allergenic if it satisfies either of the following criteria:

- a sequence identity of six or more contiguous amino acids with a known allergen;
- a minimum of 35% sequence similarity over a window of 80 amino acids with a known allergen.

Although these approaches have led to the discovery of many new allergens, they are found to be neither specific nor sensitive, and did not gain much traction with clinical scientists.

Eventually, more sophisticated methods for assessing the allergenic potential of protein sequences were developed, including the likes of SVMs, *k*-Nearest-Neighbour (kNN) classifiers, and wavelet transforms for assessing potential allergenicity of newly introduced proteins. The kNN classifier is a non-parametric density estimation technique for classifying objects based on nearest neighbors in the feature space. Here, a sequence is grouped based on the majority vote of its neighbors, and is assigned to the class most

Published by Woodhead Publishing Limited, 2013

common among its *k* nearest neighbors. Wavelet transform is a signal processing method originating from several fields including engineering, physics, and mathematics. It is commonly used for multi-resolution analysis and local feature extraction of moving signals. The method decomposes a signal into its space and scale components, and processes information based on the amplitude of the signal as well as where and when the signal occurred. Given the rising concerns of allergy-related problems, it should also be expected that many more advanced methods will appear in time to come.

Web resources: Protein allergenicity predictors

1. AlgPred
   http://www.imtech.res.in/raghava/algpred/
2. AllerHunter
   http://tiger.dbs.nus.edu.sg/AllerHunter/
3. APPEL
   http://jing.cz3.nus.edu.sg/cgi-bin/APPEL
4. SDAP
   http://fermi.utmb.edu/SDAP/

8.3 Bibliography

1. Tetko, I.V., Bruneau, P., Mewes, H.W., Rohrer, D.C. and Poda, G.I. (2006) Can we estimate the accuracy of ADME-Tox predictions? *Drug Discov. Today* **11**: 700–7.
2. Gardiner, S.J. and Begg, E.J. (2006) Pharmacogenetics, drug-metabolizing enzymes, and clinical practice. *Pharmacol. Rev.* 58: 521–0.

Published by Woodhead Publishing Limited, 2013

3. Palm, K., Stenberg, P., Luthman, K. and Artursson, P. (1997) Polar molecular surface properties predict the intestinal absorption of drugs in humans. *Pharma. Res.* **14**: 568–71.
4. Lipinski, C.A. (2000) Drug-like properties and the causes of poor solubility and poor permeability. *J. Pharmacol. Toxicol. Methods* **44**: 235–49.
5. Ghose, A.K., Viswanadhan, V.N. and Wendoloski, J.J. (1999) A knowledge-based approach in designing combinatorial or medicinal chemistry libraries for drug discovery. 1. A qualitative and quantitative characterization of known drug databases. *J. Comb. Chem.* **1**: 55–68.
6. Oprea, T. (2000) Property distribution of drug-related chemical databases. *J. Comput. Aided Mol. Des.* **14**: 251–64.
7. Wenlock, M.C., Austin, R.P., Barton, P., Davis, A.M. and Leeson, P.D. (2003) A comparison of physicochemical property profiles of development and marketed oral drugs. *J. Med. Chem.* **46**: 1250–6.
8. Congreve, M., Carr, R., Murray, C. and Jhoti, H. (2003) A 'rule of three' for fragment-based lead discovery? *Drug Discov. Today* **8**: 876–7.
9. Hou, T., Wang, J., Zhang, W., Wang, W. and Xu, X. (2006) Recent advances in computational prediction of drug absorption and permeability in drug discovery. *Curr. Med. Chem.* **13**: 2653–67.
10. Moda, T.L., Torres, L.G., Carrara, A.E. and Andricopulo, A.D. (2008) PK/DB: database for pharmacokinetic properties and predictive *in silico* ADME models. *Bioinformatics* **24**: 2270–1.
11. Wessel, M.D., Jurs, P.C., Tolan, J.W. and Muskal, S.M. (1998) Prediction of human intestinal absorption of

Published by Woodhead Publishing Limited, 2013

drug compounds from molecular structure. *J. Chem. Inf. Comput. Sci.* **38**: 726–35.

12. Wegner, J.K., Fröhlich, H. and Zell, A. (2004) Feature selection for descriptor based classification models. 2. Human intestinal absorption (HIA). *Chem. Inf. Comput. Sci.* **44**: 931–9.
13. Agatonovic-Kustrin, S., Beresford, R. and Yusof, A.P. (2001) Theoretically derived molecular descriptors important in human intestinal absorption. *J. Pharmaceut. Biomed. Anal.* **25**: 227–37.
14. Xue, Y., Li, Z.R., Yap, C.W., Sun, L.Z., Chen, X., et al. (2004) Effect of molecular descriptor feature selection in support vector machine classification of pharmacokinetic and toxicological properties of chemical agents. *J. Chem. Inf. Comput. Sci.* **44**: 1630–8.
15. Klopman, G., Stefan, L.R. and Saiakhov, R.D. (2002) A computer model for the prediction of intestinal absorption in human. *Eur. J. Pharm. Sci.* **17**: 253–63.
16. Norinder, U., Osterberg, T. and Artursson, P. (1999) Theoretical calculation and prediction of intestinal absorption of drugs in humans using MolSurf parametrization and PLS statistics. *Eur. J. Pharm. Sci.* **8**: 49–56.
17. Fujiwara, S., Yamashita, F. and Hashida, M. (2002) Prediction of Caco-2 cell permeability using a combination of MO-calculation and neural network. *Int. J. Pharm.* **237**: 95–105.
18. Ajay, Bemis, G.W. and Murcko, M.A. (1999) Designing libraries with CNS activity. *J. Med. Chem.* **42**: 4942–51.
19. Clarke, D.E. (1999) Rapid calculation of polar molecular surface area and its application to the prediction of transport phenomena. 2. Prediction

Published by Woodhead Publishing Limited, 2013

of blood-brain barrier penetration. *J. Pharm. Sci.* **88**: 815–21.

20. Grüneberg, S., Stubbs, M.T. and Klebe, G. (2002) Successful virtual screening for novel inhibitors of human carbonic anhydrase: strategy and experimental confirmation. *J. Med. Chem.* **45**: 3588–602.
21. Mekori, Y.A. (1996) Introduction to allergic diseases. *Crit. Rev. Food Sci. Nutr.* **36**: S1–18.
22. FAO/WHO (2003) *Codex principles and guidelines on foods derived from biotechnology.* Joint FAO/WHO food standards programme, Rome, Italy.
23. Nieuwenhuizen, N.E. and Lopata, A.L. (2005) Fighting food allergy: current approaches. *Ann. N. Y. Acad. Sci.* **1056**: 30–45.
24. Li, G.B., Issac, P. and Krishnan, A. (2004) Predicting allergenic proteins using wavelet transform. *Bioinformatics* **20**: 2572–8.
25. Hileman, R.E., Silvanovich, A., Goodman, R.E., Rice, E.A., Holleschak, G., et al. (2002) Bioinformatic methods for allergenicity assessment using a comprehensive allergen database. *Int. Arch. Allergy Immunol.* **128**: 280–91.
26. Stadler, M.B. and Stadler, B.M. (2003) Allergenicity prediction by protein sequence. *FASEB J.* **17**: 1141–3.
27. Zorzet, A., Gustafsson, M. and Hammerling, U. (2002) Prediction of food protein allergenicity: a bioinformatic learning systems approach. *In Silico Biol.* **2**: 525–34.
28. Soeria-Atmadja, D., Zorzet, A., Gustafsson, M.G. and Hammerling, U. (2004) Statistical evaluation of local alignment features predicting allergenicity using supervised classification algorithms. *Int. Arch. Allergy Immunol.* **133**: 101–12.
29. Cui, J., Han, L.Y., Li, H., Ung, C.Y., Tang, Z.Q., et al. (2007) Computer prediction of allergen proteins from

Published by Woodhead Publishing Limited, 2013

sequence-derived protein structural and physicochemical properties. *Mol. Immunol.* **44**: 514–20.

30. Saha, S. and Raghava, G.P.S. (2006) AlgPred: prediction of allergenic proteins and mapping of IgE epitopes. *Nucleic Acids Res.* **34**: W202–9.
31. Björklund, A.K., Soeria-Atmadja, D., Zorzet, A., Hammerling, U. and Gustafsson, M.G. (2005) Supervised identification of allergen-representative peptides for in silico detection of potentially allergenic proteins. *Bioinformatics* **21**: 39–50.
32. Sutton, B.J. and Gould, H.J. (1993) The human IgE network. *Nature* **366**: 421–8.
33. Gould, H.J., Sutton, B.J., Beavil, A.J., Beavil, R.L., McCloskey, N., et al. (2003) The biology of IGE and the basis of allergic disease. *Annu. Rev. Immunol.* **21**: 579–628.
34. Fiers, M.W., Kleter, G.A., Nijland, H., Peijnenburg, A.A., Nap, J.P., et al. (2004) Allermatch, a webtool for the prediction of potential allergenicity according to current FAO/WHO Codex alimentarius guidelines. *BMC Bioinformatics* **5**: 133.
35. Gendel, S.M. (1998) The use of amino acid sequence alignments to assess potential allergenicity of proteins used in genetically modified foods. *Adv. Food Nutr. Res.* **42**: 45–62.
36. Gendel, S.M. (2002) Sequence analysis for assessing potential allergenicity. *Ann. N. Y. Acad. Sci.* **964**: 87–98.
37. Silvanovich, A., Nemeth, M.A., Song, P., Herman, R., Tagliani, L., et al. (2006) The value of short amino acid sequence matches for prediction of protein allergenicity. *Toxicol. Sci.* **90**: 252–8.
38. Ho, J., MacDonald, K.S. and Barber, B.H. (2002) Construction of recombinant targeting immunogens incorporating an HIV-1 neutralizing epitope into

Published by Woodhead Publishing Limited, 2013

sites of differing conformational constraint. *Vaccine* **20**: 1169–80.

39. Guo, J., McIntosh, R.S., Czarnocka, B., Weetman, A.P., Rapoport, B., et al. (1998) Relationship between autoantibody epitopic recognition and immunoglobulin gene usage. *Clin. Exp. Immunol.* **111**: 408–14.

Published by Woodhead Publishing Limited, 2013

9

Vaccine adjuvant informatics

DOI: 10.1533/9781908818416.123

Abstract: The design of new molecular entities (NME) is a highly combinatorial science due to the huge array of diverse protein targets and the large chemical search space. The virtual library approach allows us to rapidly screen large libraries of compounds to identify virtual hits, which can then be purchased or synthesized, and verified experimentally. An adjuvant is an agent that is added to vaccines to enhance immune response and induce protection. It is included in the cocktail of almost all existing subunit vaccines together with antigenic peptide sequences. A wide variety of adjuvants are currently in use, including oil emulsions, aluminum salts, and a variety of small molecule compounds. In this chapter, we discuss the use of the virtual combinatorial library approach, using molecular modeling software, in the design of small molecule adjuvants with desirable pharmacokinetic properties and "drug-likeness."

Key words: virtual combinatorial library, virtual library design, new molecular entities, molecular modeling, chemical file format.

Published by Woodhead Publishing Limited, 2013

9.1 Virtual combinatorial library

The design of new molecular entities (NME) is a highly combinatorial science due to the huge array of diverse protein targets and the large chemical search space. It has been estimated that approximately 250 000 natural proteins exist, while the number of real organic compounds with molecular weight of <2000 Daltons is greater than 10^{60}. The virtual library approach allows us to rapidly screen large libraries of compounds to identify virtual hits, which can then be purchased or synthesized, and verified experimentally. This method can help minimize redundancy or maximize the number of discovered true leads by optimizing a library's diversity or similarity to a target. Virtual combinatorial library design usually begins with the explicit enumeration of all molecular variants within appropriate chemical spaces. Two approaches are commonly used to elaborate molecules:

- Markush techniques which attach a list of alternative functional groups to variable sites on a common scaffold;
- chemical transforms which specify part of the reacting molecules that undergo chemical transformations and the nature of these transformations.

The resultant libraries are then optimized for molecular diversity or similarity using molecular descriptors such as chemical composition, chemical topology, 3D structures and functionality, or drug-likeness using heuristic rules to detect ADME/Tox deficiencies.

Published by Woodhead Publishing Limited, 2013

Resources: Chemical library visualization and analysis tools

1. CLEVER
   http://datam.i2r.a-star.edu.sg/clever/
2. CORINA
   http://www.molecular-networks.com/
3. Converter
   http://www.accelrys.com/

9.2 Chemical file formats

A variety of chemical file formats currently exist. Some formats, such as MOL (and MOL2), Structure Data Format (SDF), and Crystallographic Information File (CIF), are ASCII-based files which encode the chemical structure in three-dimensional space. In general, the three-dimensional structures provided are the products of a geometry optimization, and thus the structures are in the lowest energy conformation. Most programs, however, can recognize freely rotatable bonds in these structures and thus produce multiple conformations on the fly. With the exception of MOL2 format, these structures lack the requisite atomic charges required for accurate docking studies, and thus processing of the ligands is required prior to docking studies.

Other formats, such as Simplified Molecular Input Line Entry Specification (SMILES), International Chemical Identifier (InChI), and SYBYL Line Notation (SLN), are ASCII-based files which provide structures as strings based on atom connectivity, and require an interpreter to convert the information into a three-dimensional structure; however,

Published by Woodhead Publishing Limited, 2013

string-based notations are remarkably convenient to process when doing substructure searches and comparisons as well as generating new libraries. SDF libraries may also incorporate string-based notations such as SMILES to aid in searching and sorting.

It is important to note that, although ligand libraries are readily available, it is always a good idea to check the structures for any errors. This may include fixing bond lengths and angles, atom types, and charges. In some cases, a chemical entity is in its salt form, and thus it may be necessary to remove the unnecessary cations and/or anions prior to docking studies.

9.3 Considerations for virtual library design

Several factors must be taken into account when building a virtual chemical library for small molecule design. The first and foremost consideration is that the chemical structures must have desirable pharmacokinetics in terms of absorption, distribution, metabolism, excretion, and toxicity (ADME/Tox). For the most part, Lipinski's "rule of five" provides an adequate set of guidelines for selecting drug-like compounds in terms of ADME. Other physicochemical properties have also been commonly used in the in silico design of small molecules. An example is the topological polar surface area (TPSA), which is a measure of the entire molecular surface divided by the number of polar atoms. Another such property is ligand charges. Partial atomic charges are often calculated for ligands in order to reflect the distribution of electron density around a particular molecule. Empirical and semi-empirical calculations are commonly used to account for ligand charges in molecular docking simulations. Although

Published by Woodhead Publishing Limited, 2013

ab initio methods are also available, they are more time-consuming and generally unsuitable for large ligand libraries. Most molecular modeling software includes packages for calculating partial charges. Examples of empirical and semi-empirical force fields used to calculate ligand charges include Gasteiger-Marsili charges, AMBER, MMFF, and AM1-BCC.

It is also useful to remove compounds with undesirable physicochemical properties on the basis of functional groups which are known to be reactive, or known to create false positives by indiscriminate binding. For example, acid halides (R-C(O)X) are very reactive functional groups that quickly hydrolyze to carboxylic acids (R-CO_2H), and therefore are of little use in docking studies. Functional groups such as rhodanine (2-thioxo-4-thiazolidinone) are notorious for non-selective binding to proteins. Thus, such compounds should be excluded from a ligand library prior to screening. The substructure filters for Pan Assay Interference Compounds (dubbed PAINs) by Baell and Holloway provide one such way for removing ligands which contain undesirable functional groups.

9.4 Bibliography

1. Jónsdóttir, S.O., Jørgensen, F.S. and Brunak, S. (2005) Prediction methods and databases within chemoinformatics: emphasis on drugs and drug candidates. *Bioinformatics* **21**: 2145–60.
2. Klebe, G. (2006) Virtual ligand screening: strategies, perspectives and limitations. *Drug Discov. Today* **11**: 580–94.
3. Agrafiotis, D.K., Lobanov, V.S. and Salemme, F.R. (2002) Combinatorial informatics in the post-genomics era. *Nat. Rev. Drug Discov.* **1**: 337–46.

Published by Woodhead Publishing Limited, 2013

4. Leach, A.R., Bradshaw, J., Green, D.V., Hann, M.M. and Delany, J.J. 3rd. (1999) Implementation of a system for reagent selection and library enumeration, profiling and design. *J. Chem. Inf. Comput. Sci.* **39**: 1161–72.
5. Lobanov, V.S. and Agrafiotis, D.K. (2002) Scalable methods for the construction and analysis of virtual combinatorial libraries. *Combin. Chem. High-Throughput Screen.* **5**: 167–78.
6. Livingston, D.J. (2000) The characterization of molecular structures using molecular properties. A survey. *J. Chem. Inf. Comput. Sci.* **40**: 195–209.
7. Brown, R.D., Hassan, M. and Waldman, M. (2000) Combinatorial library design for diversity, cost efficiency, and drug-like character. *J. Mol. Graph. Model.* **18**: 427–37.
8. O'Donovan, C., Apweiler, R. and Bairoch, A. (2001) The human proteomics initiative (HPI). *Trends Biotechnol.* **19**: 178–81.
9. Bohacek, R.S., McMartin, C. and Guida, W.C. (1996) The art and practice of structure-based drug design: a molecular modelling perspective. *Med. Res. Rev.* **16**: 3–50.
10. Lipinski, C.A. (2000). Drug-like properties and the causes of poor solubility and poor permeability. *J. Pharmacol. Toxicol. Methods* **44**: 235–49.
11. Hou, T., Wang, J., Zhang, W., Wang, W. and Xu, X. (2006) Recent advances in computational prediction of drug absorption and permeability in drug discovery. *Curr. Med. Chem.* **13**: 2653–67.
12. Ghose, A.K., Viswanadhan, V.N. and Wendoloski, J.J. (1999) A knowledge-based approach in designing combinatorial or medicinal chemistry libraries for drug discovery. 1. A qualitative and quantitative characterization of known drug databases. *J. Comb. Chem.* **1**: 55–68.

Published by Woodhead Publishing Limited, 2013

13. Oprea, T. (2000) Property distribution of drug-related chemical databases. *J. Comput. Aided. Mol. Des.* **14**: 251–64.
14. Wenlock, M.C., Austin, R.P., Barton, P., Davis, A.M. and Leeson, P.D. (2003) A comparison of physicochemical property profiles of development and marketed oral drugs. *J. Med. Chem.* **46**: 1250–6.
15. Congreve, M., Carr, R., Murray, C. and Jhoti, H. (2003) A 'rule of three' for fragment-based lead discovery? *Drug Discov. Today* **8**: 876–7.
16. Song, C.M. and Tong, J.C. (2009) Recent advances in computer-aided drug design. *Brief Bioinform.* **10**: 579–91.
17. Gasteiger, J. and Marsili, M. (1978) A new model for calculating atomic charges in molecules. *Tetrahedron Lett.* **19**: 3181–4.
18. Cornell, W.D., Cieplak, P., Bayly, C.I., Gould, I.R., Merz, K.M., et al. (1995). A second generation force field for the simulation of proteins, nucleic acids, and organic molecules. *J. Am. Chem. Soc.* **117**: 5179–97.
19. Halgren, T.A. (1996) Merck molecular force field. I. Basis, form, scope, parameterization, and performance of MMFF94. *J. Comp. Chem.* **17**: 490–519.
20. Jakalian, A., Jack, D.B. and Bayly, C. I. (2002) Fast, efficient generation of high-quality atomic charges. AM1-BCC model: II. Parameterization and validation. *J. Comput. Chem.* **23**: 1623–41.
21. Baell, J.B. and Holloway, G.A. (2010) New substructure filters for removal of pan assay interference compounds (PAINS) from screening libraries and for their exclusion in bioassays. *J. Med. Chem.* **53**: 2719–40.

Published by Woodhead Publishing Limited, 2013

Index

Published by Woodhead Publishing Limited, 2013

Published by Woodhead Publishing Limited, 2013

Published by Woodhead Publishing Limited, 2013

Published by Woodhead Publishing Limited, 2013

Published by Woodhead Publishing Limited, 2013

Lightning Source UK Ltd.
Milton Keynes UK
UKOW030623040713

213159UK00002B/108/P